THE PROMISE

THE PROMISE

AN INTRODUCTION TO THE HISTORY OF MEDICINE

KOUROSH NAZARI, M.D.

Universal Publishers
Irvine • Boca Raton

The Promise: An Introduction to the History of Medicine

Copyright © 2019 Kourosh Nazari. All rights reserved.
No part of this publication may be reproduced, distributed, or transmitted in any form or by any means, including photocopying, recording, or other electronic or mechanical methods, without the prior written permission of the publisher, except in the case of brief quotations embodied in critical reviews and certain other noncommercial uses permitted by copyright law.

Universal Publishers, Inc.
Irvine • Boca Raton
USA • 2019
www.universal-publishers.com

ISBN: 978-1-62734-270-4 (pbk.)
ISBN: 978-1-62734-271-1 (ebk.)

Typeset by Medlar Publishing Solutions Pvt Ltd., India

Cover design by Ivan Popov

Publisher's Cataloging-in-Publication Data

Names: Nazari, Kourosh, author.
Title: The promise : an introduction to the history of medicine / Kourosh Nazari.
Description: Irvine, CA : Universal Publishers, 2019.
Identifiers: LCCN 2018965328 | ISBN 978-1-62734-270-4 (paperback) | ISBN 978-1-62734-271-1 (ebook)
Subjects: LCSH: Medicine--History. | Medicine, Ancient. | Medical sciences. | Physician and patient. | Patients--Care. | BISAC: MEDICAL / History. | MEDICAL / Physician & Patient.
Classification: LCC R131.N39 2019 (print) | LCC R131 (ebook) | DDC 610.9--dc23.

TABLE OF CONTENTS

Introduction .... *vii*

1. The Great Observer 1
2. The Best Showman on Earth 15
3. Two Persian Princes 25
4. Purification of Medicine of Eastern Influence 35
5. Enlightenment 49
6. Pasteurization of Medicine 65
7. The German Precision 77
8. The Age of Fleming 89
9. Two American Tycoons and Two Brothers 103
10. From Barber to Surgeon 117
11. Wars and The Great Leap of Medicine 133
12. Medicine and Statesmen 147
13. American Health Care 161
14. The 21st Century and the Era of Copy Paste Medicine, Marketing, and Financial Engineering 177

15. Global Health Care Financing.. 189
16. Seeking Balance Between Hippocrates
    and Modern Forces 199

Select Bibliography *211*
About the Author *217*

INTRODUCTION

Medicine has been a part of human development and societal advancement since the beginning of time. The earliest form of medicine was practiced by women when *Homo sapiens* evolved from *Homo erectus*. Women delivered their own babies and cared for them and raised them. Anyone who has experienced a birth of a child can attest to the fact that childbirth definitely is a form of medical practice. Mothers today, as mothers throughout the history of mankind, can detect when something is wrong with their children better than anyone with advanced medical training.

Early observations and experiences of the human condition were passed down to the next generation. Unfortunately, the treatment for many of those ailments was unsatisfactory or ineffective. More importantly, the causes of those ailments were mostly attributed to bad spirits or demons. The treatments for many ailments were to keep the bad spirits away by practicing rituals and activities which did not alter the course of the disease. However, certain ailments are self-limiting, meaning they get better without any actions, thus giving credence to many therapies and practices which were of little use.

Medicine evolved and became structured when early physician philosophers wrote down the conditions they observed and organized the body of information which was available with the observation of many suffering patients. Ophthalmology and cough disorders are prominent in early medical texts. Through the ages, the understanding of the underlying causes of many disorders were identified with scientific research, and, eventually, effective scientific treatments were developed.

This book will chronicle the voyage of medicine from the early days of human history to today's medicine by highlighting individuals and events that brought us the medicine of the 21st century. Today's medical knowledge and practice have shown great promise and certain deadly habits which should be addressed and dealt with to fulfill its ultimate goal: to serve the patient. Patients are the beneficiaries of medical advances, but they were also the subject of some cruel treatments by the medical community. Some of the harm done to patients was unintentional and some was by design. Thankfully, those outrageous acts against patients were rare and rightfully condemned by the wider medical community.

Currently, medical education is largely tilted toward scientific knowledge with less emphasis on philosophy and history. The poetry side of medicine has been de-emphasized in the new Information Age. Medicine has shifted too far toward data and science, and the patient has become a data point rather than an individual.

The history of medicine is rarely taught in medical schools. This author did not receive a single hour of medical history lecture to appreciate the course of medicine and its triumphs and shortcomings through the centuries. This book attempts to provide an introduction of important figures and events in medicine to the reader. The emphasis of this book is on history and the art of medicine rather than the science of medicine. It is important to realize how we arrived at this point of medicine and critically analyze the current state of medicine. Medicine is better appreciated if the practitioners learn from the past, and not just its scientific breakthroughs but also its humanity and the ethics which strengthened through the centuries with intermittent breakdowns of its ethos. Medicine is an art which produces many wonders and some tragic outcomes, and its success still depends on the practitioner who should be informed and versed in medicine's history.

Chapter 1

The Great Observer

Medicine and the healing of man have been an integral part of human evolution and history. Every phase of the human story has involved healing and caring for the infirmed. The basic idea of medicine is caring for the sick. Every phase of human evolution has had some form of caring and tending to the weak and nurturing the sick back to health.

Three million years ago, *Homo erectus* emerged from the low-browed, big-jawed *hominid Australopithecines*. *Homo erectus* learned to make fire, use stone as tools, and most likely developed speech. This species fanned out of Africa to Europe and Asia, and, eventually, *Homo sapiens* emerged some 150,000 to 200,000 years ago.

There is scant evidence as to how early humans treated sick members. Many early humans suffered traumatic injuries such as falls or attacks by other predatory animals. Infections were most likely anaerobic soil bacteria penetrating the skin to cause gangrene. The life span of early humans was most likely into the mid- to late twenties. Since they were hunter-gatherers, the group was constantly on the move and looking for their next meal.

There are two theories regarding how those early humans cared (or did not care) for the sick. The first theory is abandonment. Since those early humans were on the move, it was not feasible to carry around the sick and weak members of the group. The weak and sick would be abandoned so the rest of the group could move and find food to ensure the survival of the rest. Evolutionary forces would eliminate the weak and ensure the survival of the fittest. The other theory is nurturing the sick back to health. The sick member is cared for by the rest of the group until he or she is well enough to be an active member of the group.

Observing animals in the wild, I can firmly state that early humans did not neatly exhibit one or the other theory but rather a combination of both. The first physicians or healers were mothers, as is the case with most primates. Human infants take longer to become self-sufficient physically. They require maternal attention for a longer period than other species. Mothers developed caring and nurturing skills to ensure the survival of early humans. Evolutionary forces made mothers the primary healers of early humans. Most likely, if a group of early humans was predominately females, the likelihood of caring for the sick and nurturing them back to health would have been much higher than if the group was predominantly male. A good example is a pride of lions. Lionesses care for the sick and watch each other's cubs. They rarely abandon the old lionesses and share the hunt with the them.

Once humans domesticated animals around 15,000 years ago, communicable diseases started ravaging human populations and continue to do so today even after many thousands of years. Most infectious diseases, such as the common cold, had ravaged other animals before jumping to humans. Pigs introduced influenza to humans and horses gave us the rhinovirus, the common cold.

Tuberculosis and smallpox were introduced to humans by cattle. Predators introduced rabies and anthrax through bites.

Nature has also caused humans misery despite its ample sustenance for mankind. Notably the Ice Age—which commenced around 50,000 BC—caused famine and hardship for early humans. The evidence of medicine in the Ice Age is scant and probably very rudimentary. Anthropology has not provided solid evidence as to the nature of medical care during the Ice Age. With the end of the Ice Age and the beginning of the agricultural phase of human development around 10,000 BC, early signs of medicine began to emerge. The earliest sign of the medicine man was found in France. The 17,000-year-old cave paintings depict humans masked in animal heads performing rituals. These were most likely witch doctors or shamans doing magic on the sick to restore them back to health. Whether they were effective is up for debate, but they provided hope to the sick, which, as many patients can attest, is crucial for healing.

More important than domesticating the animal is the next evolutionary phase of human history: the agricultural era. The agricultural age not only introduced another form of food but also caused a pleasant evolutionary change in human behavior. Before this period, most humans were hunter-gatherers. They would migrate to different parts of the world for food and shelter. With farming, humans developed a bond with the area where they cultivated crops. The land was their asset and their lifeline for food. They organized themselves around these tracts of land and began to develop rules and boundaries to protect their newfound source of food. Humans evolved from the aggressive hunters who roam the plains for their next meal to conservative farmers looking for tranquility to preserve the farm and the surrounding area. Farming also provided early medicines such as tobacco and cocaine among many herbs that early medicine men used to treat the sick.

When the Ice Age ended 10,000 years ago, humans began to cultivate the land for food and used domesticated animals in daily activities. With the advent of metalworking in the Bronze Age, 6,000 years ago, farming improved and, for the first time, humans were able to harvest crops regularly. With a steady supply of crops, settlements grew and early organized societies began to take shape.

Around 3000 BC, a tract of land between two rivers, about 100 miles upriver from the Persian Gulf in modern-day Iraq, provided the first evidence of written medicine. Those early civilizations developed laws which governed the masses and, at the same time, medical conditions were written down, along with rules governing medical treatments. Since the inception of written medicine, medical practice has been intertwined with society's laws. Law and medicine have been inseparable since its inception around this period.

Hammurabi (1728–1686 BC), the king of Babylon, introduced one of the first legal codes for society. The legal code, which was discovered in Susa, Iran (displayed in Louvre) in 1901, has laws governing medical practice in those early civilizations. It includes a pay scale for physicians and a list of punitive penalties for malpractice. The physician's fees and punishments for malpractice were based on the patient's status in society. If a physician saved a lord's life, he shall get ten shekels of silver (it's pretty generous, as it is equivalent to a laborer's annual earnings). However, if he died, the physician's hand would be chopped off. If a slave died under the care of a physician, he had to replace him.

The first medical textbook, *The Treatise of Medical Diagnosis and Prognosis*, which consists of around three thousand entries on forty tablets, was discovered in Mesopotamia. Coughing disorders and eye conditions were predominant in those early texts. The liver was considered the vital organ which provided life. There were three types of healers: *asu* (physician) who utilized drugs and performed procedures; *baru* (magician) who used divine knowledge; and *ashipu*, a priest for meditation or exorcism. The patient was treated by one or all members of this professional class. A team approach was utilized as it is today to best attain the optimal outcome. People had a belief that most diseases were the result of bad spirits invading the body. Some interpreted illness as judgment or punishment. Rituals were used to ward off the bad spirit by using potions or sorcery. People did not use these magical interventions exclusively. There is evidence of more than a hundred minerals and herbs used to treat a variety of ailments. It is safe to conclude that, in Mesopotamia, a combination of prayers, sorcery, astrology, animal sacrifice, magic, herbal drugs, and surgery was used to nurture the sick back to health.

Around the same period in Egypt, there is a body of evidence that medicine was organized and practiced utilizing a combination of magic and surgery. Discovered papyrus dated around 1500 BC in Egypt discussed surgical treatment of fractures, wounds, and abscesses. Instructions regarding circumcision, maternal care, detection of pregnancy, and contraception were found on various papyri also discovered in Egypt. Contraception for the early

Egyptians consisted of insertion of pulverized crocodile feces, herbs, and honey into the vagina.

Ebers papyrus (dated 1550 BC) describes twenty-nine eye conditions, fifteen abdominal diseases, and eighteen skin ailments. There are more than 700 herbs, drugs, and animal extracts to treat these various conditions. Treatment of eye conditions and coughs are prominent in this text. *Weakness of sight* (blurred vision) and *darkness* (blindness) are extensively discussed in the text. Treatments were mostly application of ointment made of honey, animal liver extracts, bile of turtle, plants, and herbs to the eye. An example of cough remedy was to heat a mixture of fat and herbs and inhale the smoke. Another treatment written in this papyrus was a cure for baldness which consisted of a drink made from black ass testicles, as well as the penis and vulva of a black lizard. Magic and sorcery are also discussed as part of treatments for some ailments.

Medical specialists existed in Egypt as observed by Herodotus, the great Greek historian, in 500 BC. He observed that there were physicians who treated eye conditions and those who treated the head and teeth. Medical specialties were present in the early years of human civilizations, indicating the need for specialists to treat difficult conditions. Given the prominence of eye diseases in early medical texts, ophthalmologists were probably one of the early specialists. Another notable observation about medicine in those early days is the presence of female physicians which existed in Mesopotamia. Women were an integral part of early medicine from early antiquity to the period when medicine became organized in Mesopotamia.

Around 1000 BC, across the Mediterranean Sea, a new civilization was forming that shared some traits with the Egyptians but with many noticeable differences. The Greek civilization with its array of philosophers, poets, and thinkers was reshaping man's understanding of nature, science, and life. In Homer, Apollo's son Asclepius is described as a skilled healer and the God of Medicine whose male offspring became physicians and his daughters became Hygeia (hygiene) and Panacea (cure). The modern symbol of medicine with its intertwined snakes on a winged staff originated from a statue of Asclepius. The legend of Asclepius spread through Greek societies and temples dedicated to him sprouted all over Ancient Greece. These temples served as healing shrines for the sick. They would sleep in those temples and ask for health and cure from the God of Medicine. These temples served as meeting places for the sick and the merchants of health. There were no regulations or code of conduct similar to those governing medical practice in Mesopotamia. Priests would interpret the patients' dreams at the temple for clues regarding their sickness. Magicians, herbalists, and others were present to provide service to patients.

Among those merchants of health, one school of thought stood as different from others in Greek society and other civilizations before them. Sickness was always considered a divine intervention, a plague from God, or demonic forces. One practitioner from Kos rejected this supernatural explanation of sickness. He believed that disease was the disturbance of equilibrium in the body which caused disease. Restoration of the body's equilibrium would restore a patient's body back to health. Hippocrates of Kos single-handedly changed the course of medicine and practiced a novel approach to healing which has lasted to the modern day.

Hippocrates was born around 460 BC in Kos and lived for 90 years. He was named after his grandfather which was a widely practiced custom. He was trained under his father Heracleides. Kos, along with two other towns, had Asclepius temples dedicated to teaching medicine. Hippocrates had an advantage of learning from his father as well as at the local temple of Asclepius. The medicine practiced in Kos was more focused on the patient than the disease. The other centers in Cnidus were more concerned with disease. Given the influence of medical training in Kos, Hippocrates became an avid practitioner of patient-centered medicine.

Hippocrates was an avid traveler and a great teacher. He trained many physicians, which ultimately institutionalized his approach to the healing of man. His sons, Thessalus and Draco, became successful physicians in their own right. It is possible there were multiple grandsons named Hippocrates who practiced medicine, confusing later historians as to which writing belonged to Hippocrates or his descendants. His students, sons, and grandsons continued the practice of Hippocratic medicine and enhanced the art of medicine.

Hippocrates of Kos' (approximately 460–370 BC) influence on medicine is unrivaled by others in the history of medicine. His most important contribution was his code of conduct. In early Greek society, there were no regulations of medical practice like the Code of Hammurabi in Mesopotamia. Hippocrates' initiative to have a strict code of conduct for himself, his students, and practitioners of his style of medicine distinguished them from magicians, sorcerers, herbalists, and other practitioners. He insisted on professionalism by exhibiting honesty, empathy, calmness, and a well-kempt appearance. He advocated that physicians should keep the best interest of the patient in mind and thus gain the patient's confidence and trust. Physicians should be friends of the sick.

One way to gain a patient's trust was by foretelling the future course of the disease or its prognosis. Given the limited knowledge of disease during that period, he encouraged observation of the patient and frequent visits to map the course of the disease. He was not an advocate for aggressive intervention even believing some interventions caused more harm than good, hence the axiom, *first do no harm* (*primum non nocere*). Observe, feel, listen to the patient before embarking on any action. Bedside medicine was introduced into the medical lexicon.

Here is a sample of Hippocrates' advice:

> One must note the following: conditions that disappear of their own accord; blisters such as come from fire, where this or that is beneficial or harmful; shapes of parts affected, kinds of motion, swelling, subsidence of swelling, sleep, wakefulness, restlessness, yawning; lose no time in acting or preventing; vomit, evacuations, spittle, mucus, coughing, belching, swallowing, hiccup, flatulence, urine, sneezing, tears, scratching, plucking or feeling (at hairs or bedding), thirst, hunger, plethora, dreams, pain, absence of pain, the body, the mind, ability to take in one's meaning, memory, voice, persistent silence.

The practice of medicine did not enjoy a widespread acceptance or admiration since there were many healers, priests, herbalists, magicians, and hucksters who were vying for a patient's time and money. When Alexander the Great was on his deathbed, it is believed he uttered the words, "I die by the help of too many physicians." Surgery, which derives its name by combining *cheiros* (hand) and *ergon* (work) to make *chirurgia*, says all we need to know about its position in those days. Surgery was considered a manual labor job with less esteem and prestige. The physician was the intellectual force which understood disease and was able to apply his judgment to nurture the sick back to health. Surgery did not enjoy a high regard in Hippocratic medicine. By discouraging unnecessary and injurious procedures on patients, Hippocratic physicians distinguished themselves from the rest of healers.

In the *Hippocratic Corpus*, which summarized his thoughts and writings, there is no reference to supernatural causes for disease. He wrote:

> It is my opinion that those who first called this disease 'sacred' were the sort of people we now call witch-doctors, faith-healers, quacks, and charlatans. By invoking a divine element they were able to screen their own failure to give treatment and so called this a 'sacred' illness to conceal their ignorance of its nature by picking their phrases carefully, prescribing purifications and magic along with many foods which were really unsuitable for the sick.

Hippocrates' belief that a patient is afflicted by an imbalance in the body and identifying the imbalance by studious observation marked a departure from other healers before him. In ancient Indian medicine, magico-religious explanations for sickness were prevalent. Thus, the sick person was treated by priests. In ancient China, the predominant belief was that sickness was a result of bad spirits invading the body. They surmised that good and bad spirits existed in the environment. The good spirits traveled in the air in an arc fashion while the evil spirits moved in a linear manner. Thus, to avoid sickness, the architecture of houses and buildings should make the travel of straight evil spirits more difficult by having hidden entrances or roofs and doors with many curves. Individuals with Chinese heritage seldom buy a house that has a straight stairway facing the front door. The reasoning is that linear, bad spirits would inhabit the house causing sickness.

By rejecting supernatural causes, exhibiting prudence by discouraging aggressive and injurious intervention, practicing the art of prognosis with serial observations combined with professionalism, the Hippocratic physicians ushered in an era of respectability and trust for the medical field. For the first time, Hippocratic physicians were able to make a good living practicing medicine full-time in most ancient Greek cities.

Hippocrates believed that good health emanated from good habits, exercise, eating well, and having a clean environment. He did not believe in magical cures. By studying the surroundings and habits of patients, as well as by asking questions, the imbalance could be recognized and diagnosed. Changing a patient's diet or daily activities was the first line of treatment followed by herbs, drugs, and last, if absolutely necessary, surgery was performed. Draining pus, setting fractures, and the cleaning of wounds were part of procedures that a Hippocratic physician would try. Phlebotomy was also tried during this era by Hippocratic physicians and then routinely practiced until the late 19th century.

The original oath is worth reading in its entirety to get a feel for what Hippocrates thought was important and why his influence on medicine is unrivaled by anyone or any inventions that followed him. He laid a timeless foundation on which the colossal medical endeavor was built on over millennia. He described the practice of medicine as an art and encouraged prudence and trust.

> I swear by Apollo the physician, and Asclepius, and Hygieia Panacea, and all the gods and goddesses, as my witnesses, that, according to my ability and judgement, I will keep this Oath and this contract:
>
> To hold him who taught me this art equally dear to me as my parents, to be a partner in life with him, and to fulfill his needs when required; to look upon his offspring as equals to my own siblings, and to teach them this art, if they shall wish to learn it, without fee or contract; and that by the set rules, lectures, and every other mode of instruction, I will impart a knowledge of the art to my own sons, and those of my teachers, and to students bound by this contract and having sworn this Oath to the law of medicine, but to no others.
>
> I will use those dietary regimens which will benefit my patients according to my greatest ability and judgement, and I will do no harm or injustice to them.

I will not give a lethal drug to anyone if I am asked, nor will I advise such a plan; and similarly I will not give a woman a pessary to cause an abortion.

In purity and according to divine law will I carry out my life and my art.

I will not use the knife, even upon those suffering from stones, but I will leave this to those who are trained in this craft.

Into whatever homes I go, I will enter them for the benefit of the sick, avoiding any voluntary act of impropriety or corruption, including the seduction of women or men, whether they are free men or slaves.

Whatever I see or hear in the lives of my patients, whether in connection with my professional practice or not, which ought not to be spoken of outside, I will keep secret, as considering all such things to be private.

So long as I maintain this Oath faithfully and without corruption, may it be granted to me to partake of life fully and the practice of my art, gaining the respect of all men for all time. However, should I transgress this Oath and violate it, may the opposite be my fate.

I firmly believe that certain values and practices are timeless of which there is no progress from. Trust, honesty, and sincerity should remain the bedrock of any practice no matter how sophisticated or the advances the field has experienced.

The patients' experience from the earliest days of medicine in Mesopotamia to Hippocrates' time changed from being the object whose soul was invaded by demons requiring magic and potions to a human who needed a friend and caretaker to find the cause of his predicament and nurture him back to health. While Hippocrates changed the approach and philosophy of medicine, the treatments did not change as much, and the outcomes probably did not improve. Hippocrates introduced humanity, empathy, professionalism, and a scientific basis to medicine, but it was short on effective treatments and improved outcomes. He defined medicine as a marriage of art and science that is still relevant today. The art of medicine (bedside manner) and the science of medicine (pathophysiology) are the yin and yang of medicine. The imbalance between these two forces prevents medicine from reaching its stated promise to help mankind. Knowledge without ethics and ethics without knowledge cannot succeed in the practice of medicine. Great physicians are those who have mastered the balance of these two forces. After 2,500 years, there are still debates and discussions regarding the art and science of medicine. The pursuit of the ultimate balance between art and science is still ongoing and it still needs perfecting.

CHAPTER 2

THE BEST SHOWMAN ON EARTH

Early human civilization started in Mesopotamia and spread east and west, along with its customs and practices which included the art of medicine. The power center shifted from Mesopotamia to Egypt and then to Ancient Greece. Along with the evolution of laws and societies, medicine also evolved along the route of human advancement. Once it arrived on the shore of a new civilization, the medicine practiced by many different tradesmen in Mesopotamia and Egypt changed significantly. The Hippocratic physician became different and separate from other classes of healers by having a uniform code of conduct and adherence to a set of guiding principles. As discussed before, it also became an exclusively male profession which lasted thousands of years until the late 19th century. Western medicine deviated from Aruvian medicine which was practiced in India and Chinese medicine.

Hippocratic physicians used some of the same herbs and medicines which were used in Mesopotamia and Egypt but introduced some scientific basis and organized and improved the practice of medicine. Greek civilization started its descent and a new power center was taking shape to the west. Medicine also traveled west along the path of civilization from Mesopotamia to Alexandria, Egypt to Athens and on to Rome.

Romans had low regard for Greek physicians. They considered them to be frauds and, on several monuments in Rome, it was engraved the old saying of Alexander the Great, "It was the crowd of physicians that killed me." Romans believed that lifestyle was the best medicine. One must be fit, exercise, and eat well to keep old age and disease away. However, the adventurous, globe-conquering Romans soon realized that a great physique was no match for enemies' swords and machetes. Physicians and surgeons were still needed.

The first contribution of Roman civilization to medicine comes courtesy of Aulus Cornelius Celsus (approximately 26 BC to 30–50 AD). Not much is known about him personally, but his writings made a great contribution to many fields such as law, philosophy, agriculture, military, and medicine, among others. Celsus' *Artes* (Book of Sciences) contained approximately twenty-one books. The eight volumes of books which described medical conditions and treatments survived.

Those eight books on medicine (known as *De Medicina*) provided the first comprehensive collection of knowledge about the practice of medicine. The first book covered diet and prevention. The second book described pathology and therapies. Book three and four discussed special treatments. Volumes five and six contained what can be characterized as pharmacology. Surgery and anatomy (skeletal) were covered in book seven and eight, respectively. He described inflammation using the four cardinal signs: heat, pain, redness, and swelling.

Celsus was a pivotal person in the early days of medicine and ensured that the knowledge Greek physicians had gained would not be lost in Roman civilization. By writing a comprehensive summary of medical knowledge at that point, he ensured the wisdom and information gained by Greek physicians would be transferred to the Roman civilization. The Roman physicians, in turn, built on those experiences and cataloged information to enhance the practice of medicine.

Celsus' contribution was very important but pales in comparison to the man from Pergamum (modern-day Bergama, Turkey). He had more influence and impact on medicine than any physician until the 10th century and probably the greatest personality ever to practice medicine. The man was none other than Claudius Galenos of Pergamum (130–210 AD) known as Galen. He was the most famous physician of his era and his influence on medicine lasted for 1,500 years.

He was born in 130 AD to a wealthy family in Pergamum. The city was part of the Roman Empire but had a distinctly Greek influence. Pergamum was built to compete with Athens for beauty and architecture. It had many of the attractions that were present in Athens, such as a colosseum where gladiators fought and an open-air theater.

Galen's father Nicon was a wealthy architect in Pergamum. He was very involved in Galen's upbringing. One theory why his father was so involved had to do with Galen's mother. She had a bad temper and was known to bite her servers and slaves if she was displeased by them. To keep little Galen away from his mother, Nicon would take Galen to the gymnasium, encouraged him to watch plays, and, most importantly, encouraged him to read.

Pergamum had a fine library that rivaled the library in Alexandria. Built in 304 BC by the King of Egypt, Ptolemy I, the library in

Alexandria was the preeminent place for learning and had the biggest collection of books. Pergamum's desire to have a library as important as the Alexandrian library irritated Ptolemy and he banned the export of papyrus to Pergamum and forbade any Egyptians from visiting the library in Pergamum. The embargo forced the people of Pergamum to invent an alternative to papyrus. They used animal skin to write their books. They perfected the craft of stretching and preparing animal skin which proved to be more durable and superior to papyrus. Soon, they exported their new form of "paper" to every corner of the Roman Empire.

His father also had an extensive collection of books. Galen studied philosophy by reading Plato and his famous student Aristotle. Astronomy and mathematics were part of his education. Reading Herodotus' writings opened his mind to new places and cultures. He loved reading and writing and was very inquisitive about a variety of subjects. He wrote a few books by the age of thirteen.

Throughout Greek society, there were many temples dedicated to Asclepius, who was the God of Medicine. These temples offered healing and a place of rest for the sick and injured. Pergamum had a grand temple of Asclepius which was considered one of the grandest buildings in town. It drew many people from all over the Roman Empire in pursuit of a cure. People would rest and relax in the temple in hopes of having a dream which was interpreted by priests—or fortune tellers or one of many assortments of "doctors"—to lead them to health.

Noble men of the town served in the temple to fulfill social service duties. Galen's father was also an attendant at this temple. One day while resting at the temple, he had a dream that Galen would be a physician. He encouraged Galen to study medicine and Galen started attending the temple of Asclepius to learn medicine. Among his teachers were Satyrus and Refinus. By hanging around the temple and observing the physicians who treated the people there, Galen learned the trade of medicine. His desire to read and learn led him to read about Hippocrates and his methods. Hippocrates' fame in medicine is in large part due to the inquisitive mind and prolific pen of Galen. Galen considered Hippocrates an accomplished and admirable physician and infused his teachings in his daily practice at the Asclepius in Pergamum.

At age nineteen, Galen's father, Nicon, passed away. Galen was a rich man and felt that he had learned as much as he could at the temple in Pergamum. He set his sights on the ultimate place of learning and science in all the world: Alexandria, Egypt. He initially traveled to the south of Greece and interacted and learned from the physicians that were practicing in other parts of the Roman Empire. He was very interested in botany and herbology and learned about different plants and their effects on different diseases.

He sailed from Greece across the Mediterranean Sea to Alexandria. When he got off the ship, he could hear many languages and see people and merchants from all over the world. Alexandria was a dynamic place. Africans, Indians, Persians, Hebrews, Arabs, and Romans made Alexandria the epicenter of trade and, more importantly, learning. The Museum, a huge structure where the library was housed with around 500,000 books, was similar to a massive, modern-day university. Philosophers, astronomers, physicians, and mathematicians were all gathered around the Museum to learn, debate, and discover the truth about their surroundings. It was a very intellectually stimulating place with its many libraries, study halls, parks, and, of course, an infinite amount of curiosity.

At the Museum, his closest friend was Ptolemy (not the king) who eventually became famous for writing *Almagest*, a summary of astronomy. Ptolemy's greatest contribution was his work on geography. Ptolemy told Galen that he wanted to map the land and the oceans. Galen wanted to map the human body. He studied human skeletons at the Museum where two human skeletons were housed—one was washed up on the shore at the Nile, the other was cleaned off by vultures. Dissection of the human body was forbidden in that era, so he learned a lot about human physiology by dissecting and studying the animal body. After nine years of studying in Alexandria, he was ready to practice medicine. He gathered his belongings and sailed back to Pergamum to use his skills and knowledge to heal others.

Upon his return to Pergamum, he started looking for opportunities to practice his skills. The temple of Asclepius was an option, but he felt that he could do more. One of his friends owned a *ludi*, a gladiator school. He was hired to treat the gladiators. This was a great opportunity for a young physician. Gladiators were mostly criminals and slaves who fought each other and animals in stadiums and, after a period, if they survived, they would go free. There were some free men among them who wanted the challenge, but mostly they were there to fulfill an obligation.

The gladiator sport was very brutal and violent. The injuries they suffered were horrendous. The animal attacks, machete cuts, and blunt force injuries with hammers presented an unfortunate set of circumstances for the gladiators, but they presented a unique learning opportunity for young Galen. Most gladiators did not survive a few years of combat. Most died in the ring. Galen practiced and perfected his craft by repairing dreadful wounds, fractures, and bleeding among others. The injuries were traumatic allowing him to sometimes see inside the body of humans. It gave him a unique view (literary) of the inner working of the human body. A gaping wound to the chest would allow Galen to see the human heart beating, injuries to the abdomen would show him internal vasculatures. A compound fracture—where the bone sticks through the skin—presented an opportunity to see muscle and tendon relationships to the bone.

After four eventful years at the gladiator school, where he invented surgical tools to aid in surgery, such as using heat to cauterize wounds, different techniques for wound dressing, and various kinds of scalpels, Galen felt he had achieved all he could in Pergamum. Not satisfied and always eager for a bigger challenge, he searched for his next stop that would match his sense of self-reverence. Where could possibly host a man as important as he was? In those days, there was only one place which was the center of power and prestige, Rome. He set out to travel to Rome to make a mark on history.

After a year on the road, Galen arrived in Rome and was fascinated by the city and its inhabitants. Rome was the center of the vast Roman Empire where commoners, freed slaves, senators, lawyers, and merchants all intermingled in the city center. The government provided free bread to the poor and government inspectors made sure merchants didn't gouge the residents for basic food supplies. They offered many forms of free entertainment for the masses to prevent riots and disorder. Some seats in the colosseum were free so people could watch the games. In the center of town, which was called the *forum*, where the government buildings were, people could listen to others giving speeches and arguing different points of view or advocate for their cause.

Cleanliness and sanitation were very important to the Romans, so they provided clean water and public bathhouses which were free to most people. The Romans believed that exercise and cleanliness was the best form of health maintenance, not the Greek physicians whom they thought brought death by medicine. People were skeptical of physicians and other forms of healthcare providers.

Galen got his first break in Rome to make a name for himself among many physicians and quacks who were providing healthcare in those days. His family's friend and old philosophy teacher Eudemeus was ill and not feeling well for a while. He summoned Galen for advice and treatment. Galen treated Eudemeus and he got better. Since many people in Rome knew Eudemeus, Galen's fame rose as others heard of how he cured Eudemeus.

Flavius Boethius, who was an important consul in Rome, asked Galen to cure his wife. Once his wife recovered from her disease, Boethius paid Galen handsomely and became his biggest fan. He introduced him to many important people in Rome and encouraged him to give lectures about his methods. He started by giving lectures and performing public vivisections, dissecting live animals for masses. His lectures, or more accurately his shows, became very popular with Romans and he became a mini-celebrity in Rome. After his fame, he would only treat the important people of Rome and his students would treat commoners. He continued writing and perfecting his approach to sick patients.

The common people didn't trust physicians because they didn't have access to good ones. Galen's fees were high and not many people could afford him. However, the affluent people did develop an acceptance and trust in physicians thanks largely to Galen's capabilities and skills. Galen's practice consisted mostly of house calls to the rich and famous. They would send a message that someone was sick and in need of Galen's services. He would arrive by a *lectica* (a kind of portable couch) with multiple assistants. As Hippocrates before him, he would ask questions and observe the patient and his immediate environment. His assistants would write down the history of the patient while Galen listened intently. He would prescribe one of his medications or perform a procedure and would leave the house by *lectica* again like a royalty.

His practice in Rome was very successful, but he was in constant quarrels with other physicians in town and belittled their methods and practices. He offered many apologies just to turn around and insult them again. After five years of being the center of medicine in Rome, he was tired of the hectic pace and constant verbal combat, he decided to leave Rome and head back to Pergamum once more.

His stay in Pergamum, however, was short-lived because Roman Emperor Marcus Aurelius summoned Galen back to Rome to be his physician and Galen served as a physician to four Roman emperors. He stayed in Rome until his death around 210 AD. During the last years of his life, he wrote and published hundreds of books and articles and his influence on medicine lasted more than a thousand years.

Hippocrates' importance is, in large part, thanks to Galen's writings and personality. Galen, as a young man studying philosophy and medicine, was very interested in Hippocrates' writings and thought the Hippocrates' method was the ideal way to practice medicine. Hippocrates' influence on Galen prompted him to write and perpetuate Hippocrates' teachings and methods, solidifying Hippocrates' place as the father of medicine. If Galen had rejected Hippocrates' methods or had found some other medical practitioner as the ideal physician, we would be talking about that person not Hippocrates as the father of medicine. If we think of Hippocrates as the god of medicine, Galen was the prophet who spread the word and teachings of Hippocrates all over the Roman Empire and subsequently the Western Christian civilization.

Galen's method of educating the masses by putting on medical shows in Rome enhanced the place of physicians in Roman society. His sense of importance, self-reverence, and showmanship permanently placed the physician as a respectable and financially rewarding trade which has lasted thousands of years. Physicians went from quacks and fakes to a respectable profession in society. The respect and admiration of physicians have endured all these centuries through many successive power centers. When the Roman Empire's power faded and ceded its influence on the East, the physician's importance endured and, when the center of power shifted back to the West, physicians still had a prominent, respectable place in society.

Galen's writings and teachings were part of medical training until the 15th century where new scientists and physicians questioned Galen's knowledge and understanding of medicine. Galen's understanding of medicine, which came from Hippocrates' writings, described sickness as the imbalance of humors (body fluids) of yellow bile, black bile, phlegm, and blood, which proved to be very inaccurate. His contribution to the practice of medicine as an art proved everlasting.

Chapter 3

Two Persian Princes

The practice of medicine in the Western world was shaped by Hippocrates and spread by Galen's teachings and writings. Galen accepted Hippocrates' interpretation as the ideal medical practice by physicians and expounded on it and spread the teachings to many corners of the Roman Empire. Until the disintegration of the Roman Empire in the 4th century, Galenistic medicine was unrivaled and unquestioned.

The Roman Empire, besieged by barbarians to the north and never-ending wars, was losing its influence and power. The power center of the Empire was shifting east. The Empire broke into two parts, Eastern (Byzantine Empire) and Western. After the fall of Rome in 410 AD, the Roman Empire reign was officially over. Emperor Constantine established Constantinople as the capital of the Byzantine Empire. His significant contribution to Western civilization was the establishment of Christianity as the official religion of the Empire.

Christianity, with its emphasis on service to mankind and helping the poor and the infirmed, provided a moral dimension to the practice of medicine. Medicine, as established by Hippocrates and advanced by Galen, was mostly an endeavor in seeking truth and enlightenment about human suffering. The code of ethics was more to make the profession respectable and lucrative, not a lifelong endeavor to serve man and gain favor in the Kingdom of God.

Churches, which were established in Rome during the second and third centuries, provided food and shelter to the poor. The first hospitals in the West grew out of churches as a result of early Christians' desire to serve mankind as Jesus of Nazareth and his disciples did. One of the early Christian converts, Fabiola, is credited with establishing one of the early hospitals in the West. She was a wealthy woman who dedicated her life to helping the poor and the sick. Her establishment was open to all and she would personally clean people's wounds, carry the sick from the street to her "hospital," and attend to them.

During the rise of Christianity, some of Galen's writings and teachings were losing influence. A physician from Alexandria, Paul of Aegina, and another writer, Oribasius, summarized most of Galen's teachings, and their work gave Galenistic medicine another life in the 600s AD. Their work was distributed in many parts of the Christian and non-Christian world. Their encyclopedia of medical knowledge helped many practitioners of medicine.

Christianity's main contribution to medicine was its moral teachings and instilling a sense of service to mankind. During the rise of Christianity, the practice of medicine was also theologized and became an orthodoxy. In parts of the Christian world, it was prohibited to question Galen's teachings. In contrast to Galen's medicine, which had philosophy as an integral part of it, medicine in the West became rigid and static. The teaching and practice of medicine became the domain of the church. The benefits of medicine were available to many, but the advancement of medical practice became stagnant. The stage was set for the next phase of medical advancement along with the rise of a new civilization to the east.

Islam, which was initially established in Arabia, soon spread through the east and west. It conquered Persia and India to the east and Maghreb and southern Spain to the west. It brought many different peoples and cultures under one tent with a common language. While the West was in the throes of the Dark Ages, the Muslim world embarked on the task of translating the texts of different disciplines from Persian, Latin, and others into Arabic. Arabic became the language of science. The West was not interested in scientific discovery and many scientists were punished in the West. Just like Alexandria before it, Baghdad became the new center of knowledge and science. During the 8th and 9th centuries, many medical texts were translated, including many of Galen's books. Hunayn Ibn Ishaq translated many of Galen's books into Arabic. One of the first hospitals in the East was established in Jundishapur in southern part of Iran. The main hospital where many scholars and scientists aspired to attend was established in Baghdad.

There were many Muslim physicians and scientists who contributed to the evolution of medicine, but two figures tower over the rest of Muslim scientists or any physician in the period of Middle Ages. One of the first true philosopher-scientist-physicians in the Muslim world was Zakariya Razi (865–925 AD). He was born in Rey, Iran, near Tehran. He was trained as a musician when he was young, but he soon realized that the life of a musician was not rewarded with a comfortable living. He pursued his next interest which was alchemy. His greatest contribution during his alchemy career was the discovery and purification of alcohol and its use in medicine.

During the early Muslim reign, scientific knowledge and discovery were encouraged by the caliphate. Baghdad was turned into the center of learning, and the center of medicine moved from Jundishapur, Persia, to Baghdad, and so did many aspiring physicians. One of those physicians who made the journey to Baghdad to hone his skills as a healer was Razi.

While in the West questioning Galen was forbidden, in the Muslim world, challenging established knowledge and questioning orthodoxy was gaining support among many scientists. The first step to scientific discovery is questioning the evidence and not accepting all facts. Up to this point, Galen's teachings had evolved very little. His methods were practiced throughout the West and East for a thousand years without much innovation. Razi broke with that Galenistic tradition and questioned Galen. While he admired Galen and studied much of his work, Razi also challenged Galen's methods and knowledge of disease. Razi's book, *Doubts About Galen* (*Shukuk ala Jalinus*), I argue is his greatest contribution to medicine.

He showed it was possible to admire someone and learn from him, while simultaneously questioning and, ultimately, rejecting thousand-year-old established "facts." He not only questioned Galen, but he also questioned Socrates and Aristotle's writings about the dichotomy of mind and body. He was a pioneer in mental health and its role in the overall well-being of the patient. It is reported that the first psychiatric hospital was established in the Muslim world to treat the mentally ill because of the idea that those suffering from mental illness were not "crazy" but rather ill and in need of care. Consequently, the first psychiatric hospital in the West was established in Spain in 1365 as a direct influence of Muslim medical practice.

It is difficult to grasp how the fortunes of the East and West have diverged and what we've read about the early centuries of the Muslim world is the opposite of what is practiced in many parts of the Muslim world today. Nowadays, while challenging science is routine in the West, it is heresy to question certain "facts" or figures in the Muslim world. It is worthwhile endeavor to introduce the spirit and the practice of questioning authority and "facts" as Razi did a thousand years ago. It is possible to admire and question any figure, authority, or thought without being labeled a deviant.

Razi was well-known in Baghdad and his fame landed him his next big break. The governor of Rey invited him back to Rey to open a hospital and practice there. After a while in Rey, Razi was ordered back to Baghdad by the Caliphate ruler to open another hospital in Baghdad. The selection of the site was very scientific. He hung raw meat in different parts of the city. The area which the meat remained unspoiled the longest was selected as the site of the new hospital.

His other contributions were to the fields of pediatrics, infectious disease, and ophthalmology. He described pupillary reaction and cataract surgery. It is still safe to say that he was a Hippocratic practitioner. He believed in science, but his approach to healing was patient-centered. "All that is written in books is worth much less than the experience of a wise physician," was Razi's advice to his students.

Later in life, he developed glaucoma and became blind. He spent the final years of his life in his native city of Rey, Iran. His books were translated into Latin and English and became influential in many medical schools in the West.

Up to the emergence of Razi, the great physicians were Hippocrates and Galen. Both men were alive during the great periods of Greek and Roman civilization. The Western world produced great thinkers and scientists. Aristotle, Plato, and Halcides, among others, flourished during those periods of history where free thinking and intellectual discourse was part of the fabric of Western societies. Philosophers like Aristotle and Plato were celebrities during their time and would travel and lecture. With the disintegration of the Roman Empire and decay of Western civilization, scientific inquiry and free thinking suffered in the West. As it is always in man's history, the inquisitive nature of humans does not die with changing rulers and strict, societal rules. The unending thirst for knowledge simply finds a new place to migrate to. The center of learning and science migrated from Greek city states to Alexandria and onto Baghdad. Razi revived the great tradition of the physician-philosopher who engages in healing while advancing metaphysical arguments and experimenting in alchemy. He paved the way for the next great Persian philosopher-physician who, in turn, questioned Razi and became a more consequential figure than Razi.

Even with Razi's great contributions to medicine, Galen was still unrivaled in medicine up to the late 10th century. Galen met his match in a young man as intelligent as he was with the same flair for self-promotion and showmanship. The man is no other than the Persian philosopher-physician Avicenna, Ibn Sina, (980–1037 AD). We know much about Avicenna from a great authority on Avicenna: Avicenna himself. He wrote an autobiography and explained his life experiences and adventures in the Persian territories. He was born near Bukhara in modern-day Uzbekistan under the Persian dynasty of

Samanids. He claimed to have the Quran memorized by the age of ten. In his early teenage years, he studied Persian and Arabic poetry and studied philosophers such as Aristotle. He read and studied *Metaphysics* by Aristotle forty times to grasp the meaning and he attempted to correct Aristotle's shortcomings.

He started the study of medicine at age sixteen. After studying philosophy, he found the practice of medicine rather easy. He excelled in the art of medicine and applied his philosophical knowledge to the practice of medicine. By age eighteen, he was a qualified physician and developed a reputation as a great healer in the capital of the Samanid dynasty. The ruler of the country, Nuh Ibn Mansur, sought Avicenna's advice regarding his illness. He recovered from what was reported as a serious illness under the care of Avicenna. This was his first great breakthrough and, as a reward for his service, he was given access to the library of the government where many books of famous scholars were stored. He practiced medicine during the day and studied in the evening into the night.

It also helped that Avicenna's father was a scholar and a high-ranking official in the Persian Samanid dynasty which encompassed many parts of Central Asia. Avicenna was exposed to science and learning at a young age and his first teacher was his father. When Avicenna was twenty-one years of age, his father died and the Samanid dynasty was deposed by Turkish troops. He decided against staying in the area and soon started his travels wandering in the Persian territories. He took his experience and gift of medicine to many places. At one point, he practiced in Rey, the birthplace of Razi.

He was a physician by day and a philosopher by night. He would gather his students and debate and explore the limits of logic, metaphysics, and astronomy, among many other subjects. Great men of history usually have the innate ability to excel and strive to be exceptional. They define the period as much as the period offers a milieu for them to be great. Avicenna lived in a tumultuous time where many wars were breaking out in Muslim lands. It was chaotic and unpredictable. The instability in the Persian empire forced Avicenna to travel to many parts of the country. In each stop, he was exposed to different diseases endemic to that area. He lectured in all his stops and had many students and patients who spread the word about Avicenna's exceptional ability to heal.

At one point, he was a fugitive of the state because of his affiliation with deposed rulers and was imprisoned for a period. It was during this time where he developed his philosophical theory of the floating man. He argued that if one imagined himself suspended in the air and not connected to his physical body, one could still be self-conscious thus the soul gives essence to the physical body.

Finally, when the political and military upheavals settled down, he was able to write many of his philosophical and medical books. His best and most consequential works were the *Book of Healing* and *The Canon of Medicine*. *The Canon of Medicine* was a complete encyclopedia of medicine from ancient times to the late 10th century written in an organized manner for generations to utilize in the practice of medicine. *The Canon of Medicine* was the standard textbook for medical education in the West until the 16th century. *The Canon* replaced the great works of Galen as the gold standard of medical education. After one thousand years, Avicenna's *Canon* eclipsed Galen's work and was consequential for many centuries.

Reading the works of Avicenna, one wonders how the times have changed and how everything can be possible in man's unpredictable story. Great civilizations can decay and decaying civilizations can resurrect. One work of Avicenna is worth reintroducing to the Muslim world, his argument for the existence of God. He set out to find the truth about God's existence through logic and reason. He arrived at the conclusion that God does exist by examining the universe as a chain of actual beings.

Avicenna died in Hamadan, Iran, at the age of fifty-seven. He wrote around 450 treaties on various subjects and roughly 240 of those treaties survived. Incidentally, the majority of his surviving work was on philosophy and forty texts were about medicine. His writings were about a variety of subjects such as psychology, astronomy, and geology, but he is best known for his contribution to medicine and less so to philosophy given the crowded field of great philosophers in the West. In the Islamic world, he is also best known for his contribution to medicine, but I would argue his philosophical teachings are needed in the Islamic world now more than ever. A revival of his contributions to Islamic philosophy would do a great deal of good to Middle Eastern societies.

The practice of medicine became an integral part of civilized societies which formed in Mesopotamia around 5,000 years ago and found its way back to the Middle East. The progress of medicine was along the road of great civilizations. It moved from Mesopotamia to Egypt and then to Greek city states, which produced Hippocrates, and the Greco-Roman world, which produced Galen. The node of scientific innovation went through Alexandria and back to its starting point in the Middle East during the Golden Era of Islam. While the West was in the throes of the Dark Ages, the Islamic world preserved the teachings of Hippocrates and Galen and expounded on those bodies of knowledge. Avicenna's *Canon of Medicine* was the great encyclopedia of medical knowledge which took years to write and complete. His work gathered information about medical knowledge from Hippocrates to Indian medicine and presented them in an organized and thorough fashion for aspiring physicians. It was the last time the Middle East would play a pivotal role in the progress of medicine. The torch of medicine was soon passed back to the great civilization which was finding its voice and intellectual vigor again. Medical advancement and the center of scientific breakthrough moved to Western Christian civilization and would stay there for the next thousand years all the way to the present day.

Chapter 4

Purification of Medicine of Eastern Influence

Once the Roman Empire collapsed and the European continent descended into chaos and decay, the Islamic culture in the East continued the tradition of medical education and advancement. Razi and Avicenna carried forward the Hippocratic and Galenic teachings and infused it with Middle Eastern practices. One notable contribution of Eastern culture was the treatment of mentally ill patients. The first institution to treat mentally disturbed patients was established in the Middle East.

After Avicenna, Middle Eastern societies failed to produce anyone to match his stature and contribution to the field of medicine. Avicenna's *Canon of Medicine* was taught in Europe until the mid-17th century. During the Dark Ages, medical practice and education in Europe were confined to religious institutions. Medicine became part of the religious duty of the followers of Christ. Traditional healing with herbs, honey, and divine prayers was combined to heal the patient back to health to serve God and fulfill a pious duty in the Kingdom of God. Medicine as a dynamic practice suffered during the Dark Ages and was diminished compared to Galen's days a thousand years before.

Medicine on the continent of Europe came back to life with the establishment of the first medical school in Salerno, Italy, in 1100 AD. The school was established by, what we might consider today, as a diversity officer's dream team: a Latin, an Arab, a Jew, and a Greek. The teachers and scholars at the Salerno school translated many of Galen's works from Greek to Latin. Medical texts by Galen and Hippocrates which were translated into Arabic were translated back to Latin along with the work of Muslim scholars and philosophers including Razi, Avicenna, and Hunayn. One notable figure who drove the translation of many of these texts was Constantinus Africanus (1020–1087).

The translations and compilation of all those texts from Hippocrates to Avicenna produced a comprehensive encyclopedia of known medicine which was more Galenic than Middle Eastern. The Salerno medical school produced the *Articella* (*Little Art of Medicine*), a book which combined Hippocrates', Galen's, and Hunayn's books and became the basis of medical revival and education on the continent. During this process, Galen became Christianized and formed the foundation in medical education in Christian medical education. Since Galen's art of medical practice included many of the Hippocratic teachings and writings, Hippocrates, by default once again, emerged as a cornerstone of medical education. No doubt, Galen became, once again, the man whom all true physicians should emulate. A physician should know Galen and practice as he practiced.

The translation movement and revival of medicine spread all over the continent with new universities dedicated to medical education opening in many cities. Universities were founded in Paris in 1110, Oxford in 1167, Montpellier in 1181, Cambridge in 1209, Padua in

1222, and Naples in 1224. Some of these universities awarded Bachelor of Medicine (MB) degrees in seven years and Medical Doctorate (MD) degrees in ten years. The medical education was based on the *Articella* and Avicenna's *Canon of Medicine* combined with lectures by professors based on those two texts and hands-on experience by observing practicing physicians.

This university education had to compete with churches and monasteries where the church was suspicious of university teachings. The hospitals in those days were Christian in spirit and practice. In those hospitals, Asclepius was replaced by saints of medicine, Damian and Cosmas. There were many saints in addition to Damian and Cosmas. Every specialty had its own saint; St. Luke for general illness, St. Artemis for genital disease, St. Anthony for erysipelas, St. Sebastian for epidemics, St. Christopher for epilepsy, St. Roch for plague, St. Blaise for goiter, St. Lawrence for back pain, St. Bernardine for lung ailments, St. Apollonia for dental disorders, and, most importantly, St. Margaret for childbirth.

The Western Christian world was beginning to come back to life after hundreds of years of stagnation and decay that provided an opening for Middle Eastern cultures to dominate the scientific and medical advancement. Knowledge and truth-seeking are innate human traits which cannot be extinguished. Usually the endeavor of experimentation and curiosity move to a place which is welcoming to the process. The Dark Ages in Europe did not provide the milieu for scientific and intellectual practice. Hence the center for learning moved to the Middle East which welcomed intellectual discourse. After the turn of the first millennium, the Middle East was engulfed in rivalry between Turks and Persians with the Turks dominating

Middle Eastern lands and bringing most parts of the Middle East under one empire, The Ottoman Empire.

A sentinel event caused Middle Eastern societies to start the long decay which has lasted up to this point: the Mongolian invasion. Baghdad ceased to be the center of learning and permanently lost its place after the Mongolian invasion in 1258. The Mongolian army destroyed many of the libraries in Baghdad and Alexandria and the Mongolian rulers were not known to foster discovery and scientific experimentations. They were a fighting machine which defeated most of the armies of the Middle East.

The West made a great leap with the invention of the printing press in the 15th century. Johannes Gutenberg's invention of the printing press separated Western civilization from the rest. Books could be mass produced and widely distributed within the continent. Knowledge traveled faster and wider. A movement started to bring the language of science back to its original tongue, Greek. Among the early scholars who started the movement was Desiderius Erasmus (1466–1536). He wrote and translated many of the original works by Hippocrates and Galen into Greek and some people considered him to be the originator of the medical renaissance in Europe. Galen's texts were now in Greek not Arabic and many scholars who followed him wrote the medical texts in the languages of Europe. In 1525, Aldine Press in Venice, which was a major printing house in Europe, published the completed works of Galen in Greek. Once again Galen, and by extension Hippocrates, became the luminaries and giants of medicine.

While Galen and Hippocrates were being rediscovered by Europeans, a concerted effort was underway to discredit Avicenna and Middle Eastern medicine. Among the critics of Avicenna was Nicolaus Leoniceno (1428–1524). He criticized the translation of the original Greek texts into Arabic which had altered names of certain drugs and plants. He insinuated that the misnaming of these compounds led to the wrong medicines being dispensed to the patients. He regarded the Arabic text as inferior and inelegant compared to the original Greek texts. He accused Avicenna of corrupting Galen's and Hippocrates' work in *Canon of Medicine*. Scholars rediscovered original Greek texts and printed them, bypassing Avicenna's *Canon of Medicine* which enjoyed unrivaled importance in practice and training in medicine up to the 15th century. The medical scholars in the 15th and 16th century claimed that they rescued and resurrected Hippocrates and Galen from the darkness and corruption by Avicenna and colleagues. By the late 16th century in Europe, medical practice was Galenic and Christian and Avicenna's influence was declining.

In Europe, the intellectual reawakening was sweeping many parts of society. Challenging intellectual authority and dogma was in vogue. The trait of a true intellectual was questioning established knowledge and rejecting it if it was not believed to be true. Reverence and loyalty to prior giants of science, medicine, or politics were considered priestly and unintellectual. The most important of these figures was the person who challenged the ultimate authority in the Middle Ages, which was the Catholic Church. His contribution is best explained in *Resurgence, America in the 21st Century* by this author.

Probably the most consequential figure in the rise of the West was the German priest, Martin Luther (1483–1546). His original plan was to become a lawyer, but his interest in religion induced him to enter a monastery and become a priest. In 1508, he was transferred to Wittenberg where he was a professor of theology. He struggled with the religion as to the purpose of it. He thought no matter how much good he did, it was not enough in the eyes of God. Reading St. Paul's Epistle to the Romans, he was relieved to read the phrase "The just shall live by faith." He interpreted St. Paul's word to mean that belief and faith in God was enough for salvation. Salvation was given by God as a gift to the believers and not conditioned on an individual's actions. Faith and faith only was needed for salvation.

Luther's doctrine of faith in God made certain Christian practices unnecessary or even harmful in his view. Fasting and other church-related ceremonies were obsolete since one could be saved pursuing faith as revealed in the Bible. Man does not need a priest to mediate between man and God. He can find God himself with the help of other sincere Christians. Luther's teachings were in contradiction of the Catholic Church's teachings and undermined its basic structure.

The event that prompted Martin Luther to challenge the Catholic Church was the practice of selling indulgences to the masses. During the crusades, the soldiers that went to liberate Jerusalem were promised salvation for their efforts on the battlefield. The idea of good deeds is rewarded in the Kingdom of God. However, certain people could not fight because of a disability or other reasons. Their way of salvation was to pay for someone to perform those good deeds. Simply put—if you can't do it, pay someone to do the good work for you. This practice was so profitable for the church that they expanded the selling of indulgences. Any bad deed performed by the followers of Catholicism can be washed away with purchasing of the indulgences sold by Catholic Church, although certain acts were not eligible for indulgence purchase such as murder. The practice became so corrupt that the church started selling indulgences for dead people. If anyone thought that their dead relative had done something wrong when they were alive, it was not too late to buy the indulgence and bestow on the dead relative salvation. Simply put, the Catholic Church monetized salvation.

In 1517, a preacher was in town of Wittenberg, Germany, to sell indulgences. Luther thought the act of monetizing sin was corrupt and contrary to Christian values. He challenged the practice of selling indulgences by posting his disputation, *The 95 Theses*, on the door of the church in Wittenberg. Thus, Martin Luther started the Protestant Reformation which significantly altered Christianity and allowed it to reform itself.

It was in this environment that another German figure (more accurately German-Swiss) would challenge the medical practice and knowledge of the day. Phillip Aureolus Theophrastus Bombastus von Hohenheim (1493–1541) shattered the accepted principles of medicine which were derived from Greek philosophers and medical practitioners.

The science of medicine was influenced by the Greek philosopher Aristotle. Aristotle argued that nature was composed of four elements: air, water, earth, and fire. His philosophy and work were very influential in Ancient Greece. Many philosophers and thinkers adopted his idea of four elements in different disciplines. Medicine also used the four substances to explain the body and health. The four elements in medicine were called humors. The four humors were blood, phlegm, black bile, and yellow bile, which corresponded with air, water, earth, and fire respectively. Health was attained when these four humors were in balance. Diet and other factors which caused an imbalance between these four humors caused sickness. The physician's duty was to investigate how these four humors were affected and restore them to equilibrium to cure the patient. Galen accepted the four humors theory of health and Razi and Avicenna propagated the same theory which was reintroduced to the West. For almost 2,000 years, this theory of health and disease held sway in the medical community.

Young Phillip was the son of a local physician in southern Austria. He studied at the local school which taught mining and metal analysis such as gold, mercury, and iron. His early exposure to mining and metals shaped his philosophy and understanding of human disease. At a young age, he left his hometown to travel and learn from experience rather than textbooks. He traveled all over Europe and attended many universities but was not impressed by any of the professors. He routinely mocked the professors' belief and practices. He was part of the wandering students who traveled and gained experience by learning from barbers and gypsies. He traveled to Russia, Egypt, Arabia, and Constantinople. Along the way, he was imprisoned by Tartars. He became an army surgeon in two wars. He wanted to understand nature and the forces which shaped humans and the environment. He found dignity in common people and was purported to say that he learned more from them than any high society professors at prestigious universities. He was Jacksonian in his practice and demeanor. He was a commoner who gained acceptance in universities, yet he rejected their science and understanding of human nature and found wisdom in common people.

Along his travels, he adopted the nickname Paracelsus, meaning above Celsus, who was an esteemed Roman medical writer in the 1st century. He considered himself above the prevailing medical knowledge which was over a millennium old by that time. He developed an alternative to the humoral theory of human health. He considered chemicals such as sulfur, salt, and mercury as components of human body. He introduced a new explanation of disease which was revolutionary and in conflict with prevailing practices. His combative demeanor and dogmatic belief in his science made him a notorious figure in the medical community. In 1524, he returned home and became a lecturer at the University of Basel in Switzerland. He caused consternation among the teaching staff by inviting people from all walks of life to attend his lectures. He started writing medical treaties and texts in German rather than Latin, just like Martin Luther. His lectures were also in German. He was compared to Martin Luther, but he rejected that comparison, considering himself a separate and important figure, not a follower of a societal trend. He remained Catholic until his death. His combative style and challenge to the medical society culminated in a defiant and rather Martin Luther like act. In 1527, he burned the bible of medical education in universities, Avicenna's *Canon*, in front of the university along with some of Galen's books. He wanted a departure from the old and a new beginning for medicine. After Paracelsus, medicine was divided and different schools of thought were in competition and combat. The Aristotle-Hippocrates-Galenic understanding of human disease which was expounded by Avicenna was successfully challenged by Paracelsus and started its demise. Galen and Avicenna lost their influence, but Hippocrates stayed relevant which has lasted up to this day. Hippocrates' emphasis on ethics and professionalism of the trade was timeless. There are certain characteristics and qualities which one cannot have progress from. Honesty, empathy, and caring for others are as relevant and important today as any other time.

Galen and Avicenna's emphasis on the scientific portion of disease and human health made them open to criticism and rejection. With new information and discovery, they became irrelevant and obsolete. Galen's understanding of medicine, which he wrote at the turn of the 1st century, after 1500 years, lost its prominence and prestige. Galen's and Avicenna's writings, which were so instrumental in medical education up to the 1500s, were not mentioned during this author's medical education in the 1990s. They have completely been removed from medical education in the 21st century. Yet Hippocrates enjoys its reverence among physicians today as it did during Galen's time in the 1st century.

Paracelsus' importance was his ability and perseverance in challenging the medical knowledge of the time. Yet his own reasoning and explanation of the human body and health was as wrong as the four humors theory and more dogmatic than the prevailing knowledge. He was definitely not the person who started scientific inquiry in medicine. His work and scientific method lacked clarity in thinking and his demeanor was not conducive to collaboration. Everyone's ideas or theses were dismissed if it did not agree with his thinking. He had followers after his death, but his legacy was not long-lived because he was proposing a theory at a time when human knowledge and discovery was about to embark on an odyssey unseen before in human history.

There were few important thinkers and discoverers who set in motion the Age of Enlightenment and scientific advances. Their discoveries did not play a role in the understanding of the human body or disease processes but ushered in a new age of knowledge. Among the scientists of the Middle Ages, Galileo (1564–1642) and Newton (1642–1727) were two of the most important. Interestingly, Newton was born on the day Galileo died. Newton studied and expounded Galileo's laws of motion and incorporated two other scientists' works, Copernicus (1473–1543) and Kepler (1571–1630), to become the undisputed giant of scientific discovery.

Another thinker in the Middle Ages, which I consider the father of modern science, was more a philosopher than a scientist: Rene Descartes (1596–1650) was a French philosopher and a mathematician. He experienced two personal tragedies in his life. His mother died when he was only a year old and his only child died when she was five. He was raised by his maternal grandmother and for college he moved around in Europe. He studied at a Jesuit College in La Fleche. During his years of writing and advocating for his views, he was careful not to challenge the church doctrine which had Aristotelian influence. Once he heard that Galileo was condemned by the church for his views on the earth and sun, he postponed the publication of his book, *The World*.

Descartes had peculiar beliefs and life habits. He would stay in bed till noon on most days. He also moved a lot, not only from city to city but also while in a city. He moved numerous times during his stay in the Netherlands. It was during his frequent moves when he wrote some of his greatest work and he wrote them in French as opposed to Latin just like Paracelsus, so the masses could read and learn from his thoughts and ideas. His great contribution to science was his ability to separate truth from certainty. In that period, truth came from the church which was heavily influenced by Aristotelian thinking. He set out to convince himself of matters which were certain. His first task was to prove that he existed, and his presence was not some dream. His conclusion was that he was thinking about a subject and seeking answers, so his act of thinking was proof that he existed beyond a reasonable doubt. It was self-evident that he existed because he was thinking. Therefore, his famous proverb, "I think, therefore I am," resonated and has been repeated through the centuries.

His method of reaching certainty was to arrive at a conclusion which was based on solid evidence and, therefore, no skeptic could question it. He proposed a method to seek certainty in his book, *Discourse on Method*:

1. Do not accept any idea which is not clear and self-evident.
2. Divide a problem into as many parts as possible to solve it.
3. Start solving problems from simple to complex.

4. Along the process, check and recheck the work to make sure there is no flaw or lapse in reasoning.

He used this method to explain human physiology. Unfortunately, his final product in explaining the human body was not as enduring as his method of arriving at a fair conclusion. He proposed that the body was governed by physics. The human body was like a machine and functioned under mechanical principles. The union of mind and body formed human beings and this union took place in the pineal gland. He proposed this sweeping idea without much evidence. His method was rigorous in theory but lacking in practice even for Rene Descartes. One devastating flaw of his thinking was that animals, since they do not think, have no souls and vivisection was, therefore, allowed. His conclusion that animals feel no pain resulted in mistreatment of animals over many years. Descartes' mechanical physiology was as wrong as the chemical explanation put forth by Paracelsus. But Descartes opened the way for further investigations to the ultimate explanation of human body which rapidly advanced from that point forward.

In *The Advancement of Learning*, Francis Bacon (1561–1626) had recommended a new science based on experimentation and observation to challenge Aristotelian science, but Descartes initiated the exercise of questioning and experimenting in a way that did not challenge the church. He firmly believed that humans should believe in God, otherwise there was no reason to be moral. He believed that humans, if presented with the truth, would behave morally as opposed to his contemporary colleague Thomas Hobbes

(1588–1679) who believed humans were sinful beings who needed to be coerced and managed.

Descartes was invited to Sweden to teach Queen Christina. The only problem was the lectures were scheduled at five in the morning during the cold winter. He was not accustomed to waking up early and the cold weather did not help. He developed pneumonia and died at the age of fifty-three. His contribution to medicine was important not for its scientific discovery but for the methodology of experimentation and discovery. He provided the space and reason to question the prevailing body of knowledge of the day in a way to enhance human understanding of the body without alienating or offending the dominating moral authority or the masses. Medicine would change, and the understanding of the human body would not be the same. The Aristotle-Galenic theory of medicine began to disappear from medical education to be replaced by many discoveries of a group of new enlightened frontiers.

Chapter 5

Enlightenment

With its roots in antiquity, the practice of medicine had so far evolved with civilizations and regions, but its core was still religio-philosophical with little science behind it. The mainstay of treatments for many ailments was bloodletting. Galen had recommended drawing blood from the same side and close to the diseased area, while Avicenna had advocated drawing blood from the opposite side of the diseased tissue. Both were completely wrong and useless by today's standards, and, in many instances, it was fatal to the patient. However, after centuries of civilization, during the 16th and 17th centuries, bloodletting techniques were hotly debated among physicians.

With Galen's writings and practices entrenched in the practice of medicine, Paracelsus, Descartes, and Bacon started their assault on the traditional practice of medicine by advocating for scientific methods and new ideas. However, their conclusions were as wrong as Galen's 1600 years earlier. Paracelsus' chemical theory of the body was as wrong as Descartes' mechanical theory of the body. Their efforts were noteworthy for their courage to challenge the accepted practices of medicine and understanding of the body but yielded scant results in changing the direction of the medical practice.

The change of medicine into a scientific discipline occurred with researchers, observers, and practitioners of medicine. The people who were involved in the daily care of patients and did not rely on theory or philosophical thinking to formulate hypotheses which lacked basic evidence. The first person who started the path of actual discovery of human physiology and anatomy was anatomist Andreas Vesalius (1514–1564).

Vesalius was born in Brussels, Belgium, and studied at the Catholic University of Leuven and eventually attended University of Padua where he studied the work of Persian physician Razi. The University of Padua had a strong tradition of human dissections. He developed an interest in cadaver dissection and, unlike other attending physicians, he did the dissections himself instead of relying on assistants. He soon realized that Galen's understanding of anatomy was not accurate. Galen's human anatomy was based on animal dissection since human dissection was not allowed in Ancient Rome. Vesalius had postulated that Galen's anatomy was not complete and inaccurate since the human body is different than many other species.

The first human dissection was performed by Italian physician Mondino de Luzzi (1270–1326) in 1315. With cadaver dissection now a part of many medical university curriculums, Vesalius had the opportunity to excel in human dissection and set about rewriting man's understanding of the human body. He openly challenged Galen's anatomy and published his groundbreaking book *De humani corporis fabrica libri septem* or *Fabrica* in 1543. *Fabrica* was a combination of manuscript and illustrations of the human body which were drawn in Venice under Vesalius' supervision. He traveled to Venice to personally supervise the drawings to ensure their accuracy.

Vesalius had the courage to put what he saw during dissection on paper and publish it making him instrumental in advancing human anatomy. The understanding of human physiology took an important and significant leap with the emergence of English physician William Harvey (1578–1657) and his first major scientific breakthrough in medicine. Harvey received his medical education from the same school as Vesalius, the University of Padua, and returned to England to practice medicine. He was a physician to kings and had a thriving medical practice in England. His contemporaries in England were philosophers Francis Bacon and Thomas Hobbes. He was a follower of Aristotelian thinking, but his discovery was purely scientific.

Until his discovery, just like Vesalius' groundbreaking work which discredited Galen's anatomy, human blood circulation was explained by Galen. Galen's explanation of blood circulation had many shortcomings, and no one had challenged it or corrected it. Galen's theory stated that blood was produced in the liver and filled the ventricles and through pores traveled from the right to the left ventricle. This theory and many of his explanations were utterly wrong by today's knowledge, but it was logical and accepted by other physicians for 1600 years. Harvey first pointed out the shortcoming of Galen's theory of circulation like the idea that blood was continuously being produced in the liver. By measuring the left ventricular output, Harvey correctly explained that so much blood, if continuously being made, would cause massive pressure inside the body. He correctly assumed that the blood circulated in the body starting from the right ventricle, traveling through the lungs back to the left ventricle, and during systole (contraction phase), the blood gets pumped through the body and returns to the right ventricle. The veins have a one-way valve which ensures the blood flows one way back to the heart. By comparison, Galen believed the active phase of the heart was during the dilation of the ventricles (called diastole) which sucked blood in.

Harvey correctly stated that the blood in the arteries flowed from the left ventricle to tissues and then transferred to the veins and, through valve function, returned to the right ventricle. He applied a tight tourniquet on a man's arm and observed that no blood was getting to the extremity. He then loosened the tourniquet enough that arteries would open but the vein would stay closed since veins are less elastic than arteries. He observed that the veins were filled with blood, hence the blood from arteries flows to the veins. He did not explain how this process happened which was later discovered. Harvey published his groundbreaking work *Exercitatio anatomica de motu cordis et sanquinis in animalibus* in 1628. Galen's influence rapidly faded after the one-two punch of Vesalius' and Harvey's discoveries. Galenistic physicians lead by Jean Riolan (1580–1657) attempted a counter-assault on Harvey and his discovery. Galenistic physicians realized that, once the circulatory system of Galen was challenged, then the whole of Galenic medicine would come under question. Most of Harvey's discoveries were later substantiated by researchers and the mechanism of the blood passing from artery to vein was discovered by the next breakthrough in medicine, the microscope.

Arguably the invention of the microscope ushered in a true scientific dimension to the practice of medicine. Before the use of a microscope, physicians deduced certain mechanisms since they could not see it at the microscopic level. For instance, Harvey used his deductive ability to postulate that the blood transferred from artery to vein, but he was not able to explain how and by which mechanism. Only a microscope could provide the definitive evidence by looking at the capillaries.

The invention of the microscope is credited to multiple people. However, there is a dispute as to who truly invented the instrument. Most literature credits the discovery of the microscope to two Dutch spectacle makers: Zacharias Janssen and his father, Hans Janssen. They assembled multiple lenses in a tube and realized that the objects in the other side of the tube appeared much larger than their actual size. Their discovery in the 1500s was more a novelty and an object of fascination rather than a scientific tool.

It was not until Antonie van Leeuwenhoek (1632–1723) refined the microscope with better-polished lenses in higher numbers and placed them in a tube would the microscope be useful to science. He used his refined microscope to see bacteria and protozoa. Medicine had moved from philosophical to gross anatomy and was entering the microscopic level. The English scientist Robert Hooke (1635–1703) worked with microscopes and produced the first great book about microscopic examination of matter. His book, *Micrographia*, contained microscopic illustrations of objects and living matter in great, vivid detail. The possibilities of microscopic examination of tissues started the laboratory phase of medicine.

Marcello Malpighi (1628–1694), an Italian scientist, used the microscope during his long career to explain anatomy and physiology and he is regarded by many to be the father of histology. He described many anatomical structures through microscopic examination which were not in line with Aristotle-Galenic medicine and had no shortage of detractors. But he insisted that microscopic anatomy was essential in the practice of medicine even if, at that time, those discoveries did not produce any benefit to the patient. He discovered capillaries which proved Harvey's early observations and further disproved Galen's theory. He was undeterred by his detractors and went on to describe a variety of structures such as taste buds, urinary tubules, and glomeruli (the filtering units of the kidneys).

The study of tissues was further enhanced by Giovanni Battista Morgagni (1682–1771), the anatomist at the University of Padua. His examination of the deceased to describe the cause of fatal illness and death spawned a new discipline, the practice of pathology. His groundbreaking work, *De Sedibus et Causis Morborum per Anatomen Indagatis* (*On the Sites and Causes of Disease*), became a must-have book for future pathologists. The examination of the dead at the anatomical and microscopic level produced immense amounts of knowledge about disease processes which led to future therapeutic discoveries.

During this Enlightenment period, scientific discoveries were rapid, but the practice of medicine and the remedies for patients were still inadequate. The practice of medicine was also changing, and new science was finding its way into daily, clinical practice. Santorio Santorio (1561–1636), another graduate of the University of Padua, contributed greatly to the evolution of medicine. He was very interested in new scientific discoveries in physics and wanted to incorporate them in his daily practice of medicine. He developed the thermometer to measure body temperature and a pendulum to measure pulse rates. His ingenious invention was a scale big enough where he could sleep, eat, and do work on it. He recorded his daily weight and noticed changes in his weight after eating, defecation, and sleep. His great contribution to medicine was this insistence on accurately recording all these measurements, thus introducing statistics to the practice of medicine. He published *De Statica Medicina* in 1614 which infused the science of mathematics into the art of medicine.

While Santorio introduced numerical record keeping for a single patient, Pierre Charles Alexandre Louis (1787–1872) is credited with introducing trials to the field of medicine. He was a French physician who treated pneumonia and tuberculosis and studied the practice of bloodletting in the treatment of pneumonia. He separated patients into different groups and performed bloodletting at different times to record its effects on the disease. Although his clinical trial had a small sample, he is credited with the introduction of comparative analysis. Incidentally, he died of tuberculosis himself and his research on bloodletting did not help him.

While the scientific area of medicine was beginning to take shape, clinical practice was rapidly changing as well. There were pioneers and thinkers who introduced some elements to the profession that are still used in medical practice and teaching today.

The Austrian physician Leopold Auenbrugger von Auenbrugg (1722–1809) devised the technique of percussion as a diagnostic technique. Likening the body to a drum, he postulated that striking the lungs with his fingers would make a sound just like a drum since the lungs have air and would sound dull if the lungs were full of water. His techniques were published in his book *Inventum Novum* (no need to translate this one, it's a rather obvious and grandiose title). His techniques were taught to this author during my training in the 1990s but has lost its place with widespread use of x-rays, ultrasounds, and CT scans.

Auenbrugg's *Inventum Novum* did not take the medical world by storm. But years later, the physician to Napoleon I, Jean-Nicolas Corvisart des Marets, popularized the percussion technique to assess lung and heart function. One of his students, René Laennec (1781–1826), became interested in assessing the lungs and heart in a more precise fashion. Laennec was five years old when his mother died of tuberculosis. His father was not able to take care of them and soon young René and his brother moved to live with his uncle. As luck would have it, his uncle was the dean of medicine at the University of Nantes. René followed the footsteps of his uncle and became a physician working in the lab of Guillaume Dupuytren (1777–1835) who became famous for devising a surgical technique to correct the contracture of the palm of the hand.

It was there where Laennec learned from Corvisart des Marets the techniques of percussion. The practice of lung auscultation was done by placing one's ear on the chest of the patient to listen to the heart and lung sounds. Laennec realized it was uncomfortable, especially for women, and not practical in every situation. He devised an instrument to have space between him and the patient. His instrument, a hollow wooden monoaural piece, would transmit the sounds of the chest to the practitioner's ear. Stethoscopes were born and have been a symbol and companion to physicians around the world for more than two hundred years. Years later, the wooden piece was replaced by a plastic tube and it became biaural. Laennec died of the same disease which afflicted his mother and many of his patients, tuberculosis. He died at the age of forty-five.

Not every invention by physicians in France during those tumultuous years of revolution and Napoleonic wars were like Dupuytren and Laennec. The famous weapon of terror—the guillotine—during the Jacobin purge was developed by none other than Doctor Joseph-Ignace Guillotin. It was used in England before, but Dr. Guillotin perfected the instrument by performing experiments on dead bodies in a hospital. He was also instrumental in passing a law which required capital punishment by "means of machine." The guillotine remained as an instrument of death until 1977.

During the era of Enlightenment, medical education consisted of mostly reading books and attending lectures by professors. Medical education changed from reading books to clinical experience because of the influence of the Dutch physician Hermann Boerhaave (1668–1738). He was a professor at University of Leiden and popularized bedside teaching. He was arguably the first great clinical bedside teacher. Students would travel from all over Europe to learn from him at bedside and his methods of teaching were carried to other great centers of medicine by his pupils. He attempted to collect and organize the known medical knowledge up to that point, just as Avicenna had done seven hundred years earlier. His books were widely read among physicians with his notable books being *Institutiones Medicae* (Medical principles) in 1708 and *Aphorisma de Cognoscendis et Curandis Morbis* (Aphorism on the Recognition and Treatment of Disease) in 1709.

Boerhaave wasn't the only one during this period who advocated for bedside medicine and the art of observation over new science. Thomas Sydenham (1624–1689), who preceded Boerhaave, stressed clinical bedside learning over books. Sydenham did not trust the new science of anatomy, dissection, and pathology. He stressed the best way to learn about diseases was to observe at the patient's bedside as Hippocrates had done two thousand years ago. Dr. Sydenham's emphasis on bedside learning had a great influence on Boerhaave. Because of these two men, bedside medicine did not lose influence even when new scientific discoveries were rapid and groundbreaking. Their emphasis on bedside learning was important because medicine is the art of bedside interaction infused with science.

The great center of medical education and discovery during the Enlightenment was undisputedly in Italy. As you have noticed, most of the great men who had great discoveries were connected and studied at the University of Padua. It is important to note the great scientist of that era in Italy was Galileo Galilei (1564–1642). His influence on scientific discovery was very influential on his peers and scientists of other disciplines. Santorio was inspired by Galileo to collect data and measure the body's temperature and weight. Malpighi and Morgagni were inspired to look at body tissues to discover the mysteries of the body as Galileo was looking through a telescope at the sky to uncover the universe's mystery. Galileo was one of those men whose presence, intellect, and vigor bent the arc of history in a new direction and brought people along an untrodden path to a new and brighter place. Soon the center of excellence in medicine would move north to France, the Netherlands, and England and, eventually, to Germany.

The most important discovery which altered disease process and produced direct, measurable benefits to mankind was not rooted in scientific discovery or associated with a physician or a university. An English woman, Lady Mary Wortley Montagu (1689–1762), is perhaps the most important non-physician of the Enlightenment years and her contribution is arguably greater than any other during that period because it produced an immediate benefit and alleviated much suffering among the masses. Lady Mary was born into privilege in England. She taught herself literature, Latin, among other subjects in her father's home library. When she was ready to marry, her father had arranged a marriage suitable for her. She rejected her father's suggestion and married Edward Wortley Montagu who was a Whig member of parliament. Montagu accepted the position of ambassadorship to the Ottoman Empire in 1716. Lady Mary accompanied her husband to Constantinople (modern-day Istanbul) and settled in for a life among the Turks. Lady Mary was very beautiful, had remarkable wit and charm, and was a prolific writer. She was very social and enjoyed learning about new cultures and people. She took a keen interest in the life of local women and accompanied them to the bathhouse among other activities. She wrote extensively about her experiences in Istanbul.

Lady Mary's beauty suffered when she contracted smallpox in England. Smallpox is a contagious disease which afflicted rich, poor, peasant, and royalty. Queen Mary of England (1662–1694) and Louis XV of France (1710–1774) died of the disease. She was fascinated and intrigued to observe a certain ritual during parties which women attended during fall in Istanbul. She wrote her friend, Sarah Chiswell, on April 1, 1717, about the experience:

A propos of distempers, I am going to tell you a thing, that will make you wish yourself here. The smallpox, so fatal, and so general amongst us, is here entirely harmless, by the invention of engrafting, which is the term they give it. There is a set of old women, who make it their business to perform the operation, every autumn, in the month of September, when the great heat is abated. People send to one another to know if any of their family has a mind to have the small-pox; they make parties for this purpose, and when they are met (commonly fifteen or sixteen together) the old woman comes with a nut-shell full of the matter of the best sort of small-pox, and asks what vein you please to have opened. She immediately rips open that you offer to her, with a large needle (which gives you no more pain than a common scratch) and puts into the vein as much matter as can lie upon the head of her needle, and after that, binds up the little wound with a hollow bit of shell, and in this manner opens four or five veins.

The Grecians have commonly the superstition of opening one in the middle of the forehead, one in each arm, and one on the breast, to mark the sign of the Cross; but this has a very ill effect, all these wounds leaving little scars, and is not done by those that are not superstitious, who choose to have them in the legs, or that part of the arm that is concealed. The children or young patients play together all the rest of the day, and are in perfect health to the eighth. Then the fever begins to seize them, and they keep their beds two days, very seldom three. They have very rarely above twenty or thirty in their faces, which never mark, and in eight days time they are as well as before their illness. Where they are wounded, there remains running sores during the distemper, which I don't doubt is a great relief to it. Every year, thousands undergo this operation, and the French Ambassador says pleasantly, that they take the small-pox here by way of diversion, as they take the waters in other countries. There is no example of any one that has died in it, and you may believe I am well satisfied of the safety of this experiment, since I intend to try it on my dear little son. I am patriot enough to take the pains to bring this useful invention into fashion in England, and I should not fail to write to some of our doctors very particularly about it, if I knew any one of them that I thought had virtue enough to destroy such a considerable branch of their revenue, for the good of mankind. But that distemper is too beneficial to them, not to expose to all their resentment, the hardy wight that should undertake to put an end to it. Perhaps if I live to return, I may, however, have courage to war with them.

Lady Mary explained the practice of inoculation in the Ottoman Empire which did not suffer as greatly from smallpox as in Europe. Upon her return to England, Lady Mary had her children inoculated by Dr. Charles Maitland and advocated for the practice. Initially, the inoculation was done on death row inmates who all survived the smallpox epidemic and were set free. Eventually, George II and his daughters were inoculated and the practice began to gain acceptance among the masses.

The next breakthrough came from the English country physician Edward Jenner (1749–1823). He practiced inoculation in his hometown of Gloucestershire. He noticed that the farmers who worked with cows did not develop smallpox. Cows contracted a similar condition called cowpox but once they infected humans, the virus was not strong enough to cause illness but produced immunity against more virulent human smallpox.

In 1796, Jenner inoculated an eight-year-old boy, James Phipps, with the cowpox pustule of dairymaid Sarah Nelmes. The boy developed a low-grade fever and recovered rapidly. Six weeks later, Dr. Jenner inoculated the boy with smallpox virus and the boy did not develop the disease or any symptoms. Jenner published his findings in 1798, *An Inquiry into the Causes and Effects of the Variolae Vaccinae*, and immediately attracted great attention and the practice of vaccination with a weaker virus spread all over Europe and America resulting in plummeting death rates caused by smallpox. In England, at the height of the smallpox epidemic, one-tenth of the population died of the disease. The practice of vaccination truly altered the course of human history and for the first time, humans conquered a biological foe.

Lady Mary's prolific writings and her energy and wit greatly contributed to the acceptance of the practice. She had a very interesting life ahead of her. She left England in 1739 to travel all over Europe because of "health reasons" which was a cover for an affair with an Italian writer. She lived with a few men on her odyssey and wrote about her experiences in Europe in letters to her daughter. Upon hearing the news of her husband's death, Edward Wortley

Montagu, she returned to England in 1761 and, the year after, she also passed away.

With the dawn of the 19th century, medicine had achieved great milestones in thinking and approach. With each scientific discovery and understanding of diseases, the old ways of thinking were unsustainable. The three philosophies which had dominated medical thinking and practice were shattered. The original Aristotle-Galenic philosophy came under intense criticism and its principles were not compatible with the new science. The two other competing philosophies, which attempted to supplant the Aristotle-Galenic philosophy, were quickly dismissed and failed to gain much traction with rapid discoveries in science. The chemical philosophy of Paracelsus was short-lived given its inaccuracy and the abrasive personality of its founder. The mechanical theory of Descartes, which also included the proposition that animals do not feel since they do not have souls, was soundly debunked by Charles Darwin's theory of evolution which showed humans were more closely associated to other animals. After the Age of Enlightenment, medicine would go wherever science led it and no one was sure where that would be. Medicine started losing its art and became more a science for good or ill.

CHAPTER 6

PASTEURIZATION OF MEDICINE

Medicine in the 17th and 18th century took a leap forward in scientific discovery. Man's knowledge of the human body and its physiology was never better than at the start of the 19th century. Vesalius and later Grey (of the famous *Grey's Anatomy*) dissected the body and described the details in very vivid and comprehensive ways. The microscope gave scientists and physicians a closer look at the body and Morgagni's postmortems of many dead bodies gave the science of medicine a great base of knowledge. However, all those discoveries did not result in better outcomes for the patients. This was the great dilemma and disappointment of the Enlightenment years. The promise of cures never materialized. Bloodletting was still common practice, while epidemics and infections raged across Europe. Kings, Queens, and their subjects died of communicable diseases.

One exception was the introduction of the smallpox vaccine, which was an improvement upon Turkish home remedies, and resulted in a marked reduction of smallpox transmission. The voodoo nature of medicine was still alive and present. Physicians understood how certain diseases functioned but lacked clear evidence or remedy to translate the newfound knowledge into effective treatments. Clinicians made strides with new techniques (percussion) and inventions (stethoscope) to better diagnose patients and give a proper prognosis (an area where Hippocrates excelled in), but treatments were still rooted in ancient medicine.

It is arguably the process of finding causes to diseases, and particularly infections such as tuberculosis and cholera, which led the revolution in the treatment of diseases. It was necessary to understand the human body in a correct fashion before taking the next step of finding cures, but the process was frustrating in the age where scientists like Galileo and Newton were explaining far more complicated matters.

It was the dawn of the 19th century where the center of medical excellence moved north to France. Italy's light in medicine was fading and France was emerging as the center of medical scientific excellence. It was the time of revolution and wars in France. France declared its independence from monarchy and religion lost its prominent position in many French institutions. The hospitals during the 19th century became less Christian and more secular and a new attitude toward novel thinking was taking shape in France. New ideas, especially the ones that broke with the past, were celebrated and welcomed in many sects of society.

In this milieu, Louis Pasteur (1822–1895) was born into a poor leather making family in Jura, France. His early education did not foretell his abilities as a scientist. His initial major was philosophy. After multiple failures at examination, he eventually received his Master of Science degree in 1845. His greatest contributions came when he spent time in the laboratory not taking examinations.

It is important to have a little perspective about the subject which Pasteur revolutionized. The etiology of disease—the process and cause of infection—was highly debated. Was the substance which caused infection spontaneously formed in the body or did it come from outside? There was some evidence of outside matters entering the body and causing it to develop infection. Observing the epidemics of the Black Death, syphilis, and smallpox among many epidemics in the Middle Ages, most clinicians and commoners believed in the contagion factor of infectious diseases. It was postulated by many scientists that it was an outside agent causing the disease. No one could decisively prove it, however, and the experiments were sometimes contradictory.

The process of putrefaction in dairy and meat was of considerable concern in those days. Some scientists believed, and eventually had research to prove, that the process of decay in dairy products and meat was spontaneous without external, foreign agents. Of course, it was possible those experiments were done in unsterile environments and bacteria found its way to the products. Using a microscope, scientists could see living organisms wiggling around and called them little animals or animalcules, but none connected those little animals to actual disease.

Pasteur's initial laboratory research was centered on the crystals of tartaric acid and its properties. His interest moved from chemistry to biology and focused on living matter rather than innate objects. He believed that most answers to biology lay in the laboratory and was confident he could solve them. He eventually was appointed a faculty in Lille. He started researching the process of fermentation, turning sugar into alcohol for wine and beer production and souring of milk. He moved to Paris four years later to continue to study the process of fermentation.

It is important to understand fermentation in beer and wine making to appreciate Pasteur's research. The process of fermentation—used in wine and beer making—was around for millennia. To make wine, grapes were crushed into must that had to be converted into wine. The process of making alcoholic beverage from the grape must consisted of adding a substance which was yeast to turn sugar into alcohol. Similarly, in beer making, the yeast was added usually to barley juice to turn the sugar into alcohol for the same effect. Originally, the yeast was thought to be a substance, not a living matter. They thought of yeast as a chemical matter which induced the production of alcohol from sugars.

Pasteur's contemporaries in France firmly believed the process of fermentation was a chemical process with the aid of a chemical product. Pasteur firmly believed fermentation was the result of a living microorganism. While in Paris, Pasteur embarked on a series of experimentations about the fermentation of sugar into alcohol. By 1861, he had convincing evidence to suggest that there was biological component of fermentation. He showed that fermentation required a living organism, brewer's yeast, to produce alcohol. He also demonstrated that sometimes these living organisms can live without oxygen and, therefore, they were anaerobic. He correctly observed that, when the yeast was exposed to air, there was less sugar fermentation in the solution. The air impeded the activity of the yeast.

His explanation of the process of fermentation did not produce a measurable effect on daily living or winemaking. Up to that point, he correctly explained the process that people were doing for many centuries. The next breakthrough was to solve the problem of souring of wine. Winemaking was a big business in France. Winemakers had to contend with losses from the souring of wine. Pasteur's effort to solve the riddle led him to a major discovery which affected millions of people and it is still relevant today.

In his laboratory, he demonstrated that different microorganisms in the winemaking process produced lactic acid instead of alcohol, which made the wine sour. He isolated the microorganism, *Mycoderma aceti*, which he concluded was responsible for souring the wine. If these microorganisms which soured the wine could be eliminated from the solution, then the wine wouldn't sour. Through a series of experiments, he discovered that heating the solution to 60° Celsius eliminated the offending microorganism and prevented the solution from going sour. Pasteurization of wine—and later milk and beer—was born. This discovery was as important for the masses as the discovery of vaccination. Spoiled food and milk were major sources of disease for people which was, effectively, eliminated by the simple process of heating the food, such as milk, which was a staple of the human diet, especially for children.

The next challenge was to solve the problem of putrefaction: the spoilage of meats and broth. It was commonly believed and accepted that spoilage was caused by organisms that spontaneously occurred. Pasteur challenged this notion that microorganisms were spontaneously generated. There were experiments by leading scientists at the time, such as Felix Pouchet, that provided evidence of spontaneous generation of microorganisms. Pasteur contended that those experiments were not devised and executed under optimal conditions. He basically questioned the accuracy and reliability of the studies. His study was simple yet convincing.

His experiment provided evidence of living organisms in the air which caused spoilage. He set up multiple flasks with a solution and heated them to sterilize them. A series of flasks with long swan necks prevented the germs in the air from entering the flask and the liquid did not spoil. However, the flasks which were exposed to air did spoil and had bacteria in them. Therefore, the experiment concluded that the organisms were present in the air and caused the spoilage of the liquid. His other experiments showed that heating the air and introducing the heated air to the solution also did not spoil the solution.

After establishing that there were microorganisms in the air that caused the putrefaction, he further expanded the experiment. His next question: Was the offending microorganism uniformly distributed in the air? He set up a series of flasks which had the liquid heated to kill the organisms and placed them in different parts of town, including some at high altitude locations. The flasks at high altitude had lower bacterial counts than the ones at lower altitudes. Therefore, the germs were not uniformly distributed in the air.

His work on fermentation and souring of wine, beer, and milk, as well as his experiments on broth putrefaction, started the germ theory of disease. He firmly demonstrated that microorganisms were responsible for causing disease and a way to prevent them. On February 19th, 1878, Pasteur triumphantly presented his arguments for the germ theory of infection in front of the French Academy of Medicine. A new discipline was introduced to the field of medicine: microbiology. After causing much misery, a potential treatment for these new "little animals" would alter the history of human race.

Pasteur's research and scientific discoveries also had a commercial dimension to them. He set out to solve problems affecting commercial interests and the byproduct of his research was beneficial to mankind. His major discovery of microorganisms being the origin of disease started with solving the souring of wine which progressed and culminated into developing milk pasteurization techniques which were and still are more vital for man.

His next challenge was chicken cholera which was devasting to the farmers in France. With the firm belief in germ theory of infections, he set out to solve the next crisis for farmers. He injected chickens with weeks-old cholera and observed: nothing happened to the chickens. Weeks later, he injected the same birds, as well as other birds without prior injections, with new cultures of cholera. He observed that the chickens that were immunized did not develop the disease as opposed to the birds that were not immunized. His experiments were similar to Jenner in England with cowpox.

Later, he devoted his time to solving anthrax which infected cattle and was highly contagious. Humans suffered but not at the epidemic levels which was affecting livestock. Ridding anthrax from cattle was also an exercise that had a monetary benefit to the owners of the livestock. Anthrax was very contagious and survived in the field for a long time even causing infections to animals that were not exposed to any infected animals. The staying power of anthrax and its ability to infect livestock quarantined from other infected animals was a puzzle for physicians. Robert Koch, an accomplished German scientist, had discovered the bacilli and the heat-resistant spores which caused the disease in the field. Pasteur, using the knowledge gained by Koch, experimented with the bacillus and developed a vaccine by attenuating the bacillus bacteria.

Just like Galen and other showmen in medicine, he staged a public demonstration of his discovery. He injected twenty-four sheep, six cows, and one goat with the attenuated vaccine he had discovered. He used a similar number of animals which he did not inject as a control group. Two weeks later, he injected the test animals with a stronger attenuated vaccine. The stage was set for his final piece of the study. Two weeks after the second injection, all animals were injected with a virulent strain of the anthrax-causing bacteria. Four days later, the sheep and the goat were all dead in the control (unvaccinated) group and the cows were sick. The injected (vaccinated) animals were all fine. His public demonstrations were a smashing success and his position as a preeminent scientist was forever sealed among his countrymen and eventually all over the world.

On the heels of his great success with anthrax and the publicity he received by performing the public study on livestock, he set out to solve a disease which affected humans: rabies. With anthrax, Pasteur learned that by attenuating the effect of the offending microorganism and injecting it into healthy living beings, immunity can develop effectively. The first step was always finding the causative microorganism and, in the laboratory, eliminate its effectiveness and not cause infection but have enough potency to develop immunity against the virulent strain. The problem with rabies was that the virus could not be seen by the microscopes which were available at that time. The rabies virus could only be seen with electron microscope which were not available to Pasteur. He spent hours in the lab, searching for the causing microorganism with no breakthrough.

Experimenting on rabbits, he was able to produce a non-virulent rabies virus. During the experimentation with rabbits, he learned about the long incubation period of the virus. He proceeded to test his new breakthrough on dogs which were the primary mode of transmission to humans through bites. He injected twenty-three dogs with a daily dose of the rabies vaccine with increasing strength for fourteen days. Nineteen dogs were the control and received no injections. Two weeks later, he exposed all dogs to rabies and none of the twenty-three immunized dogs developed the disease while thirteen of the nineteen dogs in the control group developed the disease. Once again, he was triumphant and his stature as a pioneering scientist was further enhanced.

Since rabies affected humans, doctors developed an interest in Pasteur's method of treating rabies. Rabies, Pasteur showed, had a long incubation period and, therefore, could be treated before the symptoms developed. On July 6th, 1885, Pasteur's moment arrived to try his discovery on a human. Nine-year-old Joseph Meister was bitten by a rabid dog and his doctor told the parents of the boy to try Pasteur for a possible treatment since he was the only one who had experimented with the disease. Pasteur did not pass up the opportunity to show his craft. Pasteur gave the boy a daily and increasingly virulent doses of rabies vaccine for fourteen days. The boy did not develop any reaction to the injection and did not develop any signs of rabies. He tried the same treatment on another boy and the boy did not develop the disease.

His talent for publicity and presentation of his experiments gained Pasteur continent-wide recognition. Thousands of people received the rabies treatments and his method rapidly gained acceptance. He was criticized by many for practicing medicine without proper training. Pasteur was not a physician, he was a scientist. Many other scientists believed that the treatment of humans should be done under the supervision of trained physicians. The criticism, however, did not slow his meteoric rise in fame, recognition, and adulation by the masses. He was revered by his countrymen for his accomplishments. The Institute of Pasteur was established in 1888 and he continued his work in the institute bearing his name. He died eight years later and was buried in his institute.

Pasteur's contemporaries hated him because they thought he was a publicity hound and his discoveries were designed to gain maximum recognition and attention rather than seek truth. He was in it for the fame, not scientific discovery. He was accused of making his experiments more conclusive than they were. Some scientists believed he covered some of the data which did not support his assertions. Of course, great men of history are not without controversy. He went against the prevailing view of the other scientists of his era and whether it was luck or ingenuity, he proved them wrong. His famous words were "In the field of observation, chance (or fortune) favors only the prepared mind." With his tenacious attitude, he accepted each challenge as an opportunity and made the most out of them. When little Meister arrived at his door, many would have declined the solicitation to inject a human without proper medical training. He eagerly delved into the treatment and, thankfully, produced an optimal outcome for the patient and himself.

History would have been different if his patient had suffered irrevocable damage or death. As he said, "Fortune favors only the prepared mind." Indeed, Monsieur Pasteur, indeed.

Pasteur's efforts and discoveries marked a transition in medicine. He was able to show that laboratory work and research could have a significant influence on the practice of medicine. The pioneers of medicine were usually physicians who treated patients and dabbled in philosophy and the science of the body. A non-physician's capability of providing useful information for medical practice was almost nonexistent. Pasteur single-handedly started the laboratory era of medicine. From that moment onward, the pioneers of medicine came from laboratories not from the clinical side. Physicians who wanted to make great strides in the practice of medicine had to spend time in the laboratory to make their breakthrough in their careers.

Medical education slowly incorporated laboratory work for their medical students. Experience in the laboratory became as important as bedside teaching. Great medical centers started incorporating laboratory work alongside patient care centers. The medical center of the future was not only a clinical hospital but also a robust and advanced laboratory setting.

Over the past two hundred years, the pioneers of the laboratory truly offered great breakthroughs in medicine. The basic understanding of human physiology examined under the microscope and incorporating chemical and biological substances in treatment of patients revolutionized medicine and directly impacted human longevity. For the first 5,000 years of human civilization, the practice of medicine had seen little change, and human life expectancy marginally improved from thirty to forty-five. In the last two hundred years, man's life expectancy jumped from forty-five to seventy-eight and, in some countries like Japan, life expectancies increased all the way to eighty. Pasteur was the first of this discipline to greatly contribute to this milestone for the human experience. Pasteurization of milk prevented countless children from contracting infectious diseases. His pioneering work with immunization prevented many from dying at much younger ages. Pasteur's experiments on putrefaction convinced ordinary people to heat their food thoroughly and cover the food and shield it from the pollutants in the air. His explanation of bacteria causing disease and infections—the germ theory—transformed physicians' understanding of the human disease process. His work directly led to changes in the medical field, such as Joseph Lister's (1827–1912) antiseptic techniques (more on him later). Pasteur's work started a chain of events in scientific medicine which culminated in one of the greatest discoveries in medicine in the early 20th century: the discovery of penicillin.

Chapter 7

THE GERMAN PRECISION

After Louis Pasteur's great successes and the fame which came along with his pioneering work, other nations and scientists appreciated the prestige and national pride that came from laboratory work. A nation to the east of France was vying to be the next great center of laboratory medicine. Germany's government was helpful in developing the budding field of laboratory investigation by providing funds and freedom for scientists to pursue their scientific discoveries.

Laboratory work had the greatest reward at the microscopic level. The German Industrial Revolution was a great help to the pioneers in the lab. The greatest instrument in those early days of laboratory work was the microscope. Nations and laboratories which had the best set of microscopes and equipment would have an advantage over other nations. In the laboratory, the precision of the instruments and the accuracy of the results were what separated great laboratory work from mediocre ones. Pasteur was able to achieve a lot without those great precise instruments. But what he lacked in equipment, he made up for in charisma and tenacity.

The German experience was different. They emphasized precision and accuracy. Their equipment became far superior to other laboratories in other countries and this superiority yielded better results and discoveries. In this national effort to make laboratories in

Germany superior through precise industrial production, Carl Zeiss (1816–1888) seized the opportunity.

Carl Zeiss sought an apprenticeship with Friedrich Körner (1778–1847) who was a great machinist. After four years of apprenticeship in Jena, Zeiss moved around Europe and finally settled in Jena to start a business in repairing precision instruments for the scientists who worked in the laboratory. He was very precise in repairing the instruments and, after repairing some of the microscopes, he realized he could make them better. The microscopes he initially built were cheaper than major rival manufacturers of microscopes. But Zeiss microscopes were more versatile, while less expensive, the scientists preferred them. Zeiss' microscopes were also easier for the students to use and affordable for them to buy. By making a better, versatile, and less expensive microscope, Carl Zeiss greatly contributed to the proliferation of the microscope's use and the acceptance of the instrument as part of regular medical education. Zeiss' company is still in business and makes some of the finest surgical microscopes, loupes, and optical lenses in the world.

By creating a great national emphasis on research laboratory work, incorporating microscopic physiology and anatomy into medical education, and the precision of the equipment made by people like Zeiss, Germany became the premier medical providers and researchers in the world. The center of discovery and medical breakthrough moved from France to Germany. Laboratory research work reached great heights in Germany and nations all wanted to emulate the German's success in research. The pioneers of medicine were no longer in the clinics; they were in the labs and Germany led the way.

One of the early German pioneers in medicine was Johannes Peter Müller (1801–1858). His use of the microscope and studies on sensory organs, like eyes and ears, was groundbreaking. He taught many students and inspired them to pursue investigational medicine. One of his students was Rudolf Virchow (1821–1902). Virchow was an interesting individual in those times. He was the son of a farmer. He was brilliant and found his way to a gymnasium which, in Germany, was a preparatory high school for students seeking to pursue a higher education. His aim was to become a pastor, and his thesis, titled *A Life Full of Work and Toil is not a Burden but a Benediction*, explains much of his personality and life calling. He had the work ethic of his father who was a farmer and a sense of duty and service to mankind from studying scripture. He soon came to the realization that he would not excel in the priesthood and ultimately pursued a career in medicine. He graduated from the University of Berlin in 1843.

Inspired by Müller and other scientists who were using the microscope to explain the intricacies of the human body, Virchow set out to continue in the same discipline. His work on the deceased resulted in instituting a structured approach to performing autopsies. He not only examined the gross anatomy of the dead body but proceeded to examine the microscopic level of the organs. He discovered many aspects of human anatomy after a disease affects the body such as Virchow's node which is an enlarged lymph node and indicates an early sign of malignancy. He is considered by some as the father of modern pathology.

His work on the cellular level was more consequential. He realized that cells arise out of other cells. He famously said, "Every cell stems from another cell." In his research, he discovered cancer cells by observing their pathology at the cellular level. He believed a lot of human illnesses could be found at the cellular level. His emphasis on the microscopic examination of tissues was one factor in the wide acceptance and requirement for medical students to perform microscopic examination of tissues in their studies. Histology and pathology became a standard part of medicine and medical education.

Virchow's discoveries were many, including the explanation of pulmonary thromboembolism and finding cells in connective tissue and bones. He described many substances such as myelin. His work on blood cells led to the discovery and description of leukemia. He found a link between human and animal infectious diseases; he was the first to use the term *zoonosis*. He was one of the main figures in Germany to advance the reputation of German medical science and contributed greatly to its newfound position as the leader in medical sciences.

Like many towering figures, he had some theories which were disproven with new evidence. He was hostile to the idea of the germ theory advocated by Pasteur. He thought that infections appeared because the host had already been diseased, making it available to host the infectious process. An internal malfunction at the cellular level made it susceptible and the presence of the microorganism was secondary. Although this position was somewhat correct in the case of cancer cells—where the internal malfunction causes cells to proliferate and malfunction—in the case of infections, the cells are entirely normal before the invading organism. Pasteur was correct, and the germ theory of infection was proven over time. Virchow also opposed hand washing which was advocated by Ignaz Semmelweis (1818–1865) to prevent infections. In 1847, Semmelweis showed that hand washing before procedures or examinations of patients reduced death rate.

Virchow also dismissed Charles Darwin's theory of evolution which was taking the scientific field by storm when it was published in 1858. He thought the idea of *Homo sapiens* descending from apes was ludicrous and believed it undermined the moral fabric of society. He believed it was an attack on the moral foundation of humanity. Later in life, he moderated his attitude toward evolution and natural selection by stating he wanted to see enough evidence to believe it. He thought there was not enough evidence to accept the whole notion of evolution.

Virchow's contributions were not solely in the laboratory or in the hospital. He was a social crusader. With his background in philosophy and religion, he always saw a social and moral dimension to the practice of medicine. In 1848, he was sent to upper Silesia by the Prussian government to study the outbreak of typhus which was devasting the population. He was not successful in controlling the outbreak, but he was appalled by what he saw there and the conditions that people lived in.

He believed that the poor state of their health was the result of their poor social standing. The poverty and blight were as much responsible for the epidemic as any medical factors he postulated. In his report, he concluded that the social transformation of the people would help their health status. A better environment and wealth, which he thought were taken away from them by landlords, would improve their health status. He equated health status with social status and ushered in a new medical discipline: social medicine. He articulately stated:

> Medicine is a social science, and politics is nothing else but medicine on a large scale. Medicine, as a social science, as the science of human beings, has the obligation to point out problems and to attempt their theoretical solution: the politician, the practical anthropologist, must find the means for their actual solution.

He became active in politics as a means of advancing medicine. He started a journal called *Medical Reform* and said, "Physicians are the natural advocates of the poor." His advocacy for social and welfare reforms played a key role in Otto von Bismarck's, the German Chancellor, remaking of German health care. He had a falling out with Bismarck after Virchow criticized his military budget. Bismarck was not amused with the criticism and challenged Virchow to a duel. It is said Virchow wisely declined but offered to duel with Bismarck using two sausages, one delicious and one laced with *Trichinella* larvae. The sausage duel never happened.

Another German who was also making headlines, not only in Germany but beyond, was Robert Koch (1843–1910), the physician and microbiologist who was Pasteur's rival. After obtaining his medical degree, Koch served as a surgeon in the Franco-Prussian War. During the war, anthrax was endemic and soon, with his laboratory work, he isolated the cause of anthrax and for the first time a causative organism was isolated which caused a specific disease. He realized that the spores of the microorganism which caused anthrax could stay dormant and become active later to infect humans or animals. Pasteur used Koch's discovery to develop his attenuated vaccine. It is important to note that Koch's discovery of the *Bacillus anthrasis*—the bacteria that causes anthrax—was the first time a causative organism was directly linked to a specific disease, thereby validating the germ theory of disease.

Pasteur was older than Koch and received a lot more attention for his discoveries, while Koch was still trying to make a name for himself in the new discipline of microbiology. With Koch's focus on obtaining recognition, he set out to bring order and discipline to the new science of microbiology. He introduced a set of principles must be observed in finding any infection-causing microorganism. These principles are known as Koch's Postulates.

1. The microorganism must be present in all cases of the infection.
2. The microorganism must be isolated from the host and grown in pure cultures.
3. The microorganism from the pure culture should cause the disease if introduced to healthy and susceptible animals.
4. The microorganism should be isolated from the new host and must be the same as the original microorganism which caused the infection.

He introduced this system and structure to the study of microbiology and set to grow the bacteria and other causative agents in the lab. He had superior microscopes and was able to isolate the offending agents better than other labs. He experimented with mediums to grow the bacteria. Initially, he used potato slices then used agar, a seaweed extract on a dish made by Richard Julius Petri (1852–1921).

Koch's method of isolating the causative agent of infection led to a major discovery. In 1882, he isolated the organism which had caused great suffering in mankind for ages. A disease that was rampant and hard to treat. He isolated *Mycobacterium tuberculosis* which caused tuberculosis. He presented his findings in front of the Berlin Physiological Society and was immediately catapulted to the ranks of elite scientist-physicians.

With the fame that came along with his discovery, new challenges also arose. The next year, a cholera pandemic was raging in Egypt and he was sent there to investigate and prevent the outbreak spreading to Europe. Pasteur's team headed by Pierre Paul Emile Roux (1853–1933) was also there searching for a solution. The French team's focus was on animal models, while Koch investigated the people who were infected. Today, we know that cholera commonly affects humans making animal studies fruitless. Koch was able to isolate the microorganism—*Vibrio cholerae*—and, not only did he show that the bacteria lived in the human intestine, but he also proved it was carried by contaminated water. This discovery led to public health reforms in water management and purification.

Koch and his students discovered many of the microorganisms which caused a variety of infections including, among others, pneumonia, typhoid, meningitis, syphilis, and leprosy. With the rapid discovery of all these organisms which cause infections, expectations were high that a cure for all these maladies that had bedeviled humanity for so long was around the corner. Just like Pasteur was successful in treating rabies, people expected more rapid discoveries of cures but that did not materialize.

One exception, however, was with diphtheria. A disease of the lungs that caused rapid coughing, vomiting, and sometimes suffocation. German scientists isolated the bacterium that caused diphtheria and, through multiple experimentations, an antitoxin serum was developed which was successfully given to a child in 1891. The child recovered and production of antitoxin was ramped up. The practice gained acceptance in Europe and America. The antitoxin serum had some problems; it could cause a reaction in certain patients such as fever, rash, and occasionally death. The benefits outweighed the costs, however, and the death rate caused by diphtheria was reduced.

Koch established an institute in Germany to study infectious diseases. He returned to the laboratory to find a cure for the most difficult of infections: tuberculosis. He had successfully isolated the causing microorganism. He was a step away from accomplishing the ultimate prize: finding a cure for an infectious disease which had caused such misery for the masses. In 1890, during a medical conference in Berlin, Koch announced that he had found a cure for tuberculosis. His cure stopped the growth of the *Mycobacterium* in test tubes and in vivo.

Koch received Pasteur-like recognition and honor. He was honored by the city of Berlin. Kaiser bestowed upon him the medal of Grand Cross of the Red Eagle. He was the man of the hour. He started using his secret treatment on patients. After a year and many patients receiving Koch's treatment, it proved it was not effective and sometimes even dangerous to the patients. The backlash against Koch was intense. Under pressure, he revealed the secret medicine was glycerin extracted from bacilli. He left Germany for Egypt because the fame he had engendered turned to animosity toward him. He made other mistakes which caused tuberculosis to further spread. His conclusion that animal tuberculosis could not be transferred to humans (or vice versa) was proven to be incorrect.

Some of his studies on tuberculosis were useful for other scientists who were looking for a cure. Eventually, scientists in France were able to prove that bovine tuberculosis and human tuberculosis were somewhat similar and contagious to each other. They were able to prevent transmission to humans by pasteurizing the milk. A vaccine was developed named Bacilli-Calmette-Guerin (BCG). Initially, the BCG vaccine was used on animals then eventually humans. The great breakthrough of the BCG vaccine came from the one center which Koch wanted to eclipse: The Pasteur Institute.

Koch was ultimately recognized for his research and pioneering work in microbiology. His disciples discovered many of the bacteria and microorganisms which caused a variety of infections. Germany perfected serum therapy and Koch's institute developed more antitoxins. Koch was awarded the Noble Prize for Physiology and Medicine in 1905. He was not able to eclipse Pasteur but, as a consolation prize (some would argue a higher prize), he was bestowed with the 21st-century high honor of having his own Doodle on Google.

During the 19th century, Germany contributed greatly to medicine by guiding medicine toward the microscopic level. Man's understanding of human function at the cellular level was the impetus to take medicine in a new direction. The breakthroughs were numerous during the 19th century in Germany. In addition to the gentlemen mentioned in this chapter, there were numerous other scientists who discovered many facets of how the human body functions at the microscopic level such as Leibig and Helmholtz. The collective scientific community in Germany was outstanding in pursuing the new field of medicine with vigor and dynamism. Germany at the dawn of 20th century was the undisputed center of medical innovation and discovery. Other countries which aspired to be a great medical center emulated the German model.

In the United States, the first great medical institution was modeled after Germany's institutions, which was dedicated to research and discovery. Johns Hopkins, the American philanthropist, donated the money to establish his namesake institution dedicated to research based on great German institutions. With Johns Hopkins University's success, other learning centers in the United States started emulating the Johns Hopkins model which was, essentially, the German model.

A new world was taking shape across the Atlantic that was ambitious and determined to emulate and eclipse Europe's success in many fields, medicine included. The 19th-century medicine belonged to Germany except for a few isolated talents such as Pasteur who disturbed the German monopoly of scientific discovery. With the new century, many challenges were awaiting Europe and a few miscalculations by its leaders plunged the continent into war and chaos and Europe ceased to be the center of scientific progress. That title went to the new nation to the west: the United States of America.

Chapter 8

The Age of Fleming

The 19th century was a turning point for medicine. The nature and tenor of practicing medicine changed drastically. The Aristotle-Galen approach to physiology and anatomy became absurd after numerous discoveries made in the 19th century. Pasteur, Koch, and his pupils in Germany radically changed the way disease, specifically the infectious process, was understood. The germ theory of disease was well accepted by the 20th century. The religio-philosophical school of thought lost its position in medical thinking. Medicine became more scientific and laboratory-based than ever before.

Despite all the breakthroughs and discoveries in the 19th century, the treatment of disease was still less than desirable. Vaccination against smallpox, Pasteur's immunization, and pasteurization of milk contributed greatly to effective prevention and treatment of certain infections, but a readily available treatment for most infections was not present. Koch's famous misfire and debacle with his "miracle" tuberculosis treatment humbled many scientists and reminded everyone that man's historical nemesis, infectious microorganisms, still had the upper hand.

Man's history and human civilization are intertwined with microbes. Infectious diseases have a long history and great impact on human history and man had always felt powerless. The microbes affected kings and queens as well as ordinary people. After a century of great discoveries, microbes still had the upper hand in the early 20th century as illustrated by the story of Calvin Coolidge Jr.

A nation was rising to the east of Europe which was redefining governance and the relationship of government to the people. The United States in the 1920s was a rising power with many milestones. The Wright brothers had conquered gravity by inventing flying. Electricity was redefining homes and the night. Cars were produced in great numbers and were transitioning humans from riding carriages to driving cars. The 1920s in America was an exciting time. The way humans lived was rapidly changing. The leader of this dynamic nation was none other than Silent Cal, President Calvin Coolidge (1872–1933).

President Coolidge was a modest man with few words to share with the nation, yet his governing style was principled and strong and led the nation through a great decade. He became president when President Harding died while in office and Coolidge assumed the presidency on August 3rd, 1923. After settling in the White House, the Coolidges took a family photo in the White House on June 30th, 1924. Coolidge had two sons, John, eighteen, and Calvin Jr., sixteen. By all accounts, Calvin Jr. was President Coolidge's favorite child.

After this photo, the two brothers went to the White House tennis court for a lively, competitive brotherly match. Calvin Jr. did not wear socks for this match and, during the game, he developed a blister on one of his toes. The brothers ended the match early and went inside. The blister on Calvin Jr.'s toe got worse and developed an infection. He spiked a fever and sepsis was developing.

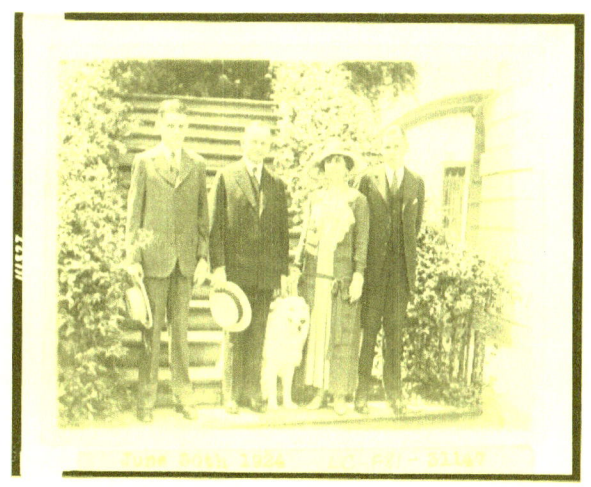

On July 3rd, 1924, Calvin was moved to Walter Reed Military Hospital and was attended by leading physicians in the country. After four days at the hospital, Calvin Jr., the son of the most powerful man in the country. died of a toe infection. On July 7th, 1924, only seven days after that happy photo in the White House, a member of the first family was dead, succumbing to a strain of bacteria. Another win for man's deadliest nemesis.

Infectious microorganisms have caused misery and death for as long as man has been on this Earth. The infection which Calvin Jr. developed was most likely caused by *Staphylococcus Aureus* which lives on human skin and can penetrate an open wound and cause an infection, sepsis, and death. It was as deadly for the Neanderthals many thousand years ago as it was in the early 20th century for *Homo sapiens*. Little had changed in combating the infection once it developed. Strides were made in prevention of infections with hand hygiene but, once an infection developed, the outcome was dependent on the body's natural defense mechanisms.

Non-communicable infectious diseases were detrimental and lethal to the individuals who developed them but did not cause mass casualty. Communicable infectious diseases were more detrimental to the individuals and the societies they affected. Communicable infectious diseases became more common and deadly when civilizations formed, animals were domesticated, and people lived in close quarters. When cities grew, and commerce developed between peoples and nations in far-flung places, the era of epidemics and pandemics started with devastating efficiency.

The Justinian Plague, which is named after Roman Emperor Justinian I, occurred in the year 541 AD. Rats from Egypt brought the plague to the capital city of Constantinople and resulted in a catastrophic loss of life. At the height of the disease, some 5,000 people died per day in Constantinople. When the epidemic ran its course, 40% of the people of Constantinople had vanished. It's estimated that 25 million people died from the disease. This episode is the first recorded outbreak of bubonic plague which is caused by the bacterium *Yersinia pestis*.

Almost 900 years later, the same plague devasted Europe in the Middle Ages. Since the cities were larger and commerce was more developed, the second outbreak of the epidemic was for the history books. The social, economic, and medical impact on the people of Europe was and still is unmatched by any event in history. In a four-year span, from 1347 to 1351, at least 75 million people died (the world population was approximately 450 million). It is estimated that more than thirty percent of the population of Europe perished in those four years. It is nicely summarized in the book *Resurgence* by this author.

It is unfortunate to mention a tragic event as a catalyst for the revival of a civilization, but one cannot deny its impact on the population of Europe. In 1347, a Genoese ship docked in Messina off the Sicilian coast. The well-wishers were horrified to see most of the people on the ship were dead and the ones living had large black boils on their bodies. The people alive on the ship had fevers, were delirious, and had black boils on their skins which oozed blood and pus, thus it was named the Black Death. Upon seeing the condition of the sailors, the ship was made to leave the port at once. However, it was too late. The disease spread throughout the continent and resulted in the death of twenty million people—a third of the population of Europe.

The disease caused by a bacillus bacterium spread from person to person through the air. People did not understand how the disease spread and widespread suffering resulted, causing people to avoid each other. Doctors refused to see their patients, neighbors stopped socializing, and people fled to the countryside. Some people believed it was a divine punishment for the sins of their society. To get rid of the plague, God's forgiveness was necessary.

The human population on Earth has been controlled and kept in check with communicable and non-communicable infectious diseases. While the most devastating pandemic was caused by a bacterium, other great communicable diseases were viral, such as the Spanish Flu of 1918, HIV, and Antonin Plague (most likely smallpox). These communicable diseases were more devastating than any war humans have waged on each other. The two most devasting wars were World War II, with approximately 50 million deaths, and the Mongolian Invasion of Persia and wider Middle East, with an estimated 30 to 40 million deaths; but both pale in comparison to what the Black Death did to Europe and the world with some estimates of more than 100 million deaths. To conquer one of these sources of the infection such as bacterial infections would be a coup for human survival and expansion.

The quest to overcome bacteria started with Pasteur. While studying anthrax bacilli, he noticed when another bacterium was added to a solution where anthrax bacilli was present, the production of additional bacilli was halted. One microorganism competed with another microorganism and deprived it of what it needed to grow and multiply. The action of one microorganism acting against another bacterium was termed *antibiosis*. The principle of living organisms acting as soldiers to destroy a more potent bacterium was the first step in the quest to produce a cure.

While Pasteur and Koch contributed greatly to the study of bacteriology, the greatest breakthrough and impact belongs to the Scottish microbiologist Alexander Fleming (1888–1955) who worked at St. Mary's Hospital in London. During World War I, Fleming worked on wounds suffered by soldiers and his focus was on the prevention of infection. He realized that certain agents killed the natural defenses of the wound without affecting the infecting bacteria. Certain widely used agents to wash the wounds resulted in promotion of infection rather than preventing it. In 1921, he had his first breakthrough by identifying *lysozyme*, which was present in tears and mucosal fluids, and destroyed certain bacteria. The lysozyme was not strong enough to kill more potent bacteria.

In 1928, one of best-timed vacations produced the greatest breakthrough in the human struggle against bacteria. Fleming was working on *staphylococci*, the same bacterium that killed Calvin Coolidge Jr. After returning from vacation, he noticed one of the Petri dishes had formed mold and the mold had destroyed the *staphylococcus* colonies. He identified the mold as *Penicillium rubrum* and published his results in 1929. Later, it was realized the correct name was *Penicillium notatum*. The publication of his paper did not cause any celebration in the medical community and actually was little noticed at the time.

Fleming's discovery was dormant until ten years later, when a team of Oxford scientists led by Howard Florey (1898–1968) and Ernst Chain (1906–1979) researched the literature for their quest in treating bacterial infections and discovered Fleming's study. With the aid of biochemist Norman Heatley (1911–2004), they produced enough of the penicillin drug to test it on animals. In 1940, the team injected eight mice with streptococci bacteria. Four were treated with penicillin. The four treated mice survived, and the four untreated mice all died. They knew they had a wonder drug.

They produced enough to treat a patient. The first person to receive penicillin was a policeman whose wound from gardening had become infected. He was given the penicillin drug and he improved remarkably, but they ran out of the penicillin and the patient eventually got worse and died. Realizing the potential for the drug, Florey approached British pharmaceutical companies about the mass production of penicillin. In the height of the greatest war humanity had seen, the British companies had other priorities. Florey traveled to the United States to mass produce the drug. In the United States, Florey and Heatley were able to mass produce the drug. With enough penicillin, Florey traveled to North Africa to test the drug on the wounded soldiers. It was a smashing success. The tide was turned, man had conquered one of its greatest enemies, bacterial infections. For this great discovery, Fleming, Florey, and Chain shared the Noble Prize in 1945.

Around the same time, German scientific laboratories were hard at work trying to discover a cure for bacterial infections. The chemical industries of Germany in the early 20th century was the gold standard in industrial engineering. Gerhard Domagk (1895–1964) was a German physician-scientist working at company called Bayer on compounds which could treat bacterial infections. He made a class of drugs called sulfa drugs derived from azo dyes. He named the first sulfa drug Protonsil which was effective against certain bacterial infections. Sulfa drugs are bacteriostatic drugs, unlike penicillin, they do not kill the bacteria, but they inhibit its growth and multiplication, allowing the body's immune system to overcome the infection. Domagk was so convinced of his new drug's efficacy that he used the drug on his own daughter for a streptococcal throat infection.

Domagk's discovery was important in starting the chemical revolution of medicine. Medicine could be made from chemical components as opposed to natural substances to treat disease. Natural substances like penicillin were difficult to mass produce, while the drugs derived from chemical components could be made in significant amounts in the laboratory. Other countries like Britain followed the German lead and made chemical drugs along the same line as sulfa drugs. The British company May and Baker developed a drug named M&B 693 which was similar to sulfa drugs to treat infection. Winston Churchill received this drug during World War II to treat a bacterial pneumonia infection while in Tunisia. It was wrongly reported that Churchill received penicillin. It was understandable that politics sometimes massages the truth to enhance the standing of a nation. Penicillin was an Anglo-American product while sulfa drugs were a German invention. In the height of World War II, in the battle between fascism and democracy, it was a better story to give the credit to the Allies as opposed to the Axis.

The politics of the two antibiotics did not end with the saga of Churchill's treatment. Sulfa drugs were banned in certain countries because of the animosity between Germany and many countries in Europe. For example, France would not allow the production of sulfa drugs, because of national pride and fear of ruining the vaccination industry which was robust in France. Domagk was awarded the Nobel Prize in Medicine in 1939 for the discovery of sulfa drugs, but he was prevented from receiving it because the Nazi government was mad at the Nobel committee for awarding the Nobel Peace Prize to the German pacifist Carl von Ossietzky in 1935. Domagk eventually received the Nobel Prize in 1947. The Allies were victorious in the struggle between fascism and democracy and the discovery of penicillin received a far higher importance in medical history textbooks. In time, penicillin became more relevant and useful in medicine as opposed to sulfa drugs. But the drug revolution, which started in the industrial-chemical complex of Germany, led to massive discoveries of various drugs to treat a multitude of diseases.

While penicillin was active against gram-positive bacteria, it had little effect on gram-negative bacteria and on *Mycobacterium tuberculosis* which had affected humanity for millennia and proved hard to treat. The breakthrough for treating tuberculosis infection came from the New World. Selman Waksman (1888–1973), a Russian immigrant to the United States, discovered an antibiotic which was effective in the laboratory but too toxic to humans, *actinomycin*. He pursued the same line of research and eventually isolated a fungus named *Streptomyces griseus*. The antibiotic extracted from the fungus, *streptomycin*, proved very effective against *Mycobacterium tuberculosis*. Later, another antibiotic, *Isoniazid*, was developed, and the combination therapy was highly effective against tuberculosis and finally effectively controlled the saga of tuberculosis infections which had claimed the lives of millions throughout history. Finally, the incidences of tuberculosis infections plummeted.

Infections and communicable diseases ravaged many civilizations before the discovery of penicillin and vaccination. When Christopher Columbus discovered the New World, the settlers managed to conquer the Americas not with guns or huge armies but with the aid of communicable diseases. Settlers brought smallpox from Europe and the native population of continental America had no immunity to combat smallpox and the disease ravaged the native population. It killed more than a third of the people on the American continent. Once they survived smallpox, measles arrived on the heel of smallpox by way of new European settlers and wiped out almost half of the population.

The trade with the New World was not a one-way route. The Europeans brought back syphilis from the New World to Europe and it spread all over Europe. From Spain, it spread to France during the war in 1493 and continued to spread all the way east to India and Japan. Incidentally, syphilis was called a different name in different regions depending who brought it. It was called Polish disease in Russia, Christian disease in Turkey, and Portuguese disease in Japan. The effects of syphilis were nowhere near as devastating as the introduction of smallpox and measles by Europeans, and malaria and yellow fever by Africans to America. Before the discovery of penicillin and vaccination, the effects of infectious diseases were devastating and civilization altering.

The decades between the 1920s and 1960s was the golden age of drug development. Various drugs were discovered to treat a variety of diseases. Hypertension, gout, malaria, and rheumatoid arthritis were among many diseases that were successfully treated with the array of new miracle drugs. Suddenly, a physician's medicine chest was full of different drugs to treat patients. Gone were the days of bloodletting, watching patients helplessly and comforting them in their dying days from preventable infections. Cortisone, which was isolated in the Mayo Clinic in the 1930s, was life-changing for patients with inflammatory diseases such as rheumatoid arthritis. The drug revolution of the early 20th century was unprecedented in human history.

All those discoveries and, more importantly, the discovery of penicillin to treat bacterial infections combined with vaccination, personal hygiene, and public sanitation efforts led to the extension of the average life expectancy. For the earliest humans, life expectancy at birth was estimated to have been around thirty years. Life expectancy in Europe around the turn of 20th century was between 40 to 45 years. After millennia of civilization, enlightenment, and great discoveries in the early 1900s, a person born in Europe could reasonably expect to reach forty. It may seem dismal compared to today's standards; but, by 1950, a mere fifty years later and the European life expectancy leaped to almost sixty years of age. It was a remarkable leap in just 50 years to reach this milestone. With the exception of the Spanish Flu in 1918, life expectancy continued its upward trajectory to reach the late seventies at the turn of 21st century. In one hundred years, humanity went from a life expectancy of forty years to almost eighty years. This milestone was due to the cumulative effect of vaccination, the triumph over bacterial infections which could affect a person from birth to death, the improvement of public sanitation efforts, and the control of chronic medical diseases.

The discovery of penicillin by Fleming and the subsequent studies and experiments done by Florey and Chain were a definite turning point for medicine and human civilization. Bacterial infections had terrorized the masses for as long as humans have been on Earth. The century prior to the discovery of penicillin was marked by great discoveries in understanding disease, specifically bacteria. But all those discoveries did not produce any great, direct benefit to mankind. Penicillin and other antimicrobials extended human life, which subsequently produced more human capital and accumulated more knowledge, and that, in turn, resulted in other discoveries and inventions in other fields.

The tenor of human civilization changed with the discovery of penicillin. One outcome was the graying of advanced societies. The distribution of people in societies shifted from young to aged. Societies also exhibited older and wiser characteristics. Younger societies tend to be more aggressive, impulsive, and compulsive as opposed to older societies which are more measured, patient, cerebral, and prudent. The wars which were fought in the 18th, 19th, and early 20th centuries were largely replaced with sporadic wars on a much smaller scale. World War I and World War II occurred during the periods where the societies of Europe and Asia were younger and had more aggression, energy, and troops. With the aging of many societies around the world, the destructive and expansive wars subsided.

After World War II, when the societies started aging with the help of antibiotics and other drugs, the major wars were small, local, and between societies with younger populations. Since World War II, the bloodiest wars have been between societies who are young. The Rwanda Genocide, the Iran and Iraq war, and the Syrian civil war occurred between societies with young populations.

The needs and political orientation of older societies changed as well. The governments became more responsive to the needs of their (now older) population and spent more time and resources to cater to them with better health care and pension. The government's expenditure shifted from a military focus to social and retirement columns. The economies of those societies changed as well. The focus was on the needs of the aged as opposed to the young, since the aged had more money to spend. Whole new industries such as retirement homes—unheard of in the beginning of the 20th century—became big business by the turn of the 21st century.

The above examples are just a few observations resulting from Fleming's discovery. Until human life expectancy changes for better or worse, these dynamics will be with us, and, therefore, this is the Age of Fleming more than any other description of the current era.

Chapter 9

Two American Tycoons and Two Brothers

During the 18th and 19th century, the practice of medicine was drastically changed. Medicine, which had been rooted in philosophy and metaphysics, changed to a scientific field like astrology and physics. The early practicing physicians were the mothers who took care of their offspring and the worthy adult members of the clan. The practitioners of medicine evolved over time during the early civilizations in Mesopotamia to become professionals whose main job was attending to the sick. The full-time physicians which were part of early civilizations were mainly religious-magic practitioners with some practical approaches. The practice of medicine was not standardized and there was no authority among civilizations to set the guidelines for the practice of medicine.

Medicine became less religious and somewhat more scientific when Hippocrates rejected the idea of illness as a curse but rather a misfortune upon those affected. He provided a guideline and set of principles to manage the profession. He was successful in influencing the early Greek physicians to adopt his principles of practice and brought respectability to the profession. The science behind what they did was not adequate or close to any logic or scientific basis compared to what physicians know today about the body and disease. Hippocrates' was fortunate to have influenced a giant in medicine centuries later to adopt his principles and teach others. Galen, the giant of medicine, was the first true international showman physician with a knack for dramatic presentations and a prolific pen.

Galen's writings and teachings formed the basis for medical education for 1,500 years. Avicenna and Razi contributed to the field of medicine but they did not alter the trajectory of medicine. They built upon Galen's writings and practices but did not fundamentally change the practice of medicine. Up until the Enlightenment era, to be a physician was to know and read Galen. During the Reformation and Age of Enlightenment, the tenor of medicine changed in radical ways. Paracelsus, Descartes, and others challenged the prevailing science of the time to usher in a new era. Paracelsus' and Descartes' explanations of disease and the human body were as wrong as Hippocrates, Galen, and Avicenna, but the taboo of criticizing the saint of medicine, Galen, was shattered.

The center of medical knowledge started in Mesopotamia moved west to Egypt and traveled north to the Greek city states and onward to Rome. With the decay of the Roman Empire and resurrection of Middle Eastern culture, the center of medicine moved back to the Middle East. The glory days of Islamic culture and medicine was eclipsed with the Renaissance in Europe. Europe came out of the Dark Ages and the nodal point of medicine and discovery moved back to Western Christian civilization. Medicine was a companion to the journey of power and civilization which oscillated between the West and the East. The resurrection of the Western Christian civilization was entirely different than other civilizations before it.

Once Europeans settled (or more accurately accommodated) their religious differences through the Thirty Years' War, the peace accord reached at Westphalia in 1648 set the stage for remarkable centuries of new discoveries, inspiring art, beautiful music production, and inventions. Medicine was reshaped along with the many fields of life that were altered for the better during those centuries.

With the aid of human dissection, the invention of microscope, and new thinking about diseases and the body, medicine was transformed. The great medical centers in Europe were first built in Italy, then moved north to France, the Netherlands, and England, and finally they came to Germany. By the turn of the 20th century, there was no doubt about the center of medical discovery and education being in Germany. France was instrumental during the 18th and 19th centuries in creating vaccines and investigative microbiology. The Pasteur Institute, established in France, was very influential in the field of microbiology. Medical discovery had moved from clinics to laboratories with the German laboratories being the gold standard at the turn of the 20th century.

A new power was rising to the west which was vying for a position on the global stage. A young nation with high aspirations and ideals was shaping up across the Atlantic Ocean. Young Theodore Roosevelt, the 26th President of the United States of America, willed the country into thinking big and having higher aspirations than dominating its own hemisphere. With the expansion of its naval forces and carving an active role for America on the world stage, he disregarded George Washington's advice to stay away from foreign entanglements and became an international player. He earned a Noble Peace Prize for brokering peace between Russia and

Japan. President Woodrow Wilson, another idealist, thrust America into the Great War during the 1910s. The unsatisfactory conclusion to World War I coupled with the war debt and the economic downturn created an atmosphere in America which fostered public regret and backlash against America's involvement in the European war. America turned inward and focused on herself.

The 1920s in America was one for the ages. The leap in living conditions and inventions was extraordinary and many of the inventions are still with us today. Cars, airplanes, electricity, refrigerators, stoves, radio, and television are just a few examples of the new products that were introduced to daily life during the 1920s. In ten years, daily living was radically altered and the people creating them were as eclectic as the new inventions. Other fields were also testing the limits of what was possible. Civil engineers and architects were building high rises never seen before or even thought possible just a few years before. Movies moved from robotic pictures to talking movies. Assembly line production was introduced, and the cost of a new car was affordable for many. The "Roaring Twenties" was an exciting time in America and the people felt that the possibilities were boundless.

In that era of inventions, discoveries, and euphoria, the practice of medicine in America was less than desirable and lacked the innovation or the prestige compared to European countries. While America was becoming a leader in manufacturing, military, and aviation, the practice of medicine in America lacked imagination, respectability, and innovation. It was a disappointment to many given all the news about new drugs, discoveries, and treatments which were taking place in Europe.

From the start of the Union, the practice and training of medicine in America was similar to the course of the nation in those early days. People were suspicious of central control and resisted rules and regulations regarding the practice of medicine. When the concept of the United States was formed, a physician was at the table. Benjamin Rush (1746–1813), the only physician signatory on the Declaration of Independence, played a significant role in shaping the new nation. He was against slavery, pro-women's education, and anti-capital punishment. He famously wrote *Medical Inquiries and Observations, Upon the Diseases of the Mind* which started the basis for psychiatry in America. Although he was active and an intellectual, he contributed little to the organization of medicine in the new country. The laws governing the practice of medicine were scant and a variety of people claimed to be able to treat patients.

This freewheeling approach had some horror stories regarding patient care and surgery. The practice of medicine in America did not have a uniformed quality and rigor which existed in Europe. However, this unregulated environment, under which the American medical system functioned, had some positive side effects. The first women to earn medical degrees in the West graduated from American medical schools. Elizabeth Blackwell (1821–1910) was a British citizen who earned a medical degree in America. She was the first woman to be awarded a Medical Doctorate degree and was followed by her sister Emily Blackwell (1826–1910). The first American woman to receive a medical degree was Lydia Folger Fowler (1823–1879). Women were able to become doctors in America before Europe allowed women to become physicians. The less regulated American medical system allowed some improvisation and experimentation which was not the case in Europe. Women were finally able to gain medical degrees.

The freewheeling medical system in America produced some welcome developments such as admission of women and minorities into medical schools but the overall landscape of medical education and practice was not sufficient for a nation aspiring to become a first-rate nation with power and prestige. Medical education was mostly a profit center for local physicians who would train prospective students. As such, there was a wide variation in experiences for the medical students. There was no standard or benchmark for all these institutions which were training medical students. The quality of the education, therefore, was very substandard in many places and the medical degrees awarded did not carry as much prestige given that the medical schools were not known for quality clinical practice or research. Medical education in Europe was mostly connected to research centers and universities and the degrees carried weight. In short, medical education in America was not uniform or high quality in many places and the degrees awarded were not highly regarded.

During the Industrial Age in Europe and in America, certain individuals amassed massive wealth which was not seen ever in human history. Throughout history, significant wealth was connected to the seat of power such as kings and princes. In America, the system allowed certain individuals to create companies which rewarded the founders' immense wealth never before seen in human history. The Industrial Age produced such a tectonic shift in human civilization that it upended many sectors of the economy and the way humans worked. It also created massive disparity in wealth distribution. Individuals with massive wealth were richer than the ruling class in America. The industrialists were euphoric over their inventions and discoveries which had revolutionized the human living experience. Henry Ford's assembly line produced affordable cars for masses. Planes were able to ferry people around the country. Alexander Graham Bell (1847–1922) invented the telephone which connected people despite great distances, and Thomas Edison (1847–1931) was able to bring light to the darkness (literally).

This era, which was called the Gilded Age, produced a few wealthy men. Among them was John D. Rockefeller (1839–1937). He rose from a modest upbringing to start an oil company which eventually controlled 90% of the refineries and oil wells in America. He was ruthless in terms of buying out competitors with unfair practices and intimidation, but it produced a hugely profitable monopoly. His company, Standard Oil, was eventually broken into thirty companies in 1911. During his time and ascent in the business world, he met a priest who advised him on investments and business. In the 1890s, Rockefeller had turned over the control of the day-to-day business of his company to others. Inspired by other tycoons of his era, he became active in philanthropy. Frederick Taylor Gates (1853–1929), the American Baptist clergyman, who had advised Rockefeller about other aspects of his business became his principle philanthropy advisor. He oversaw the distribution of more than $500 million to charities. He urged Rockefeller to spend money on medicine and education to have the most impact. Businessmen never cease to be outdone even in philanthropy. Rockefeller wanted his money spent on endeavors that would produce the most positive effects on society and receive maximum recognition, which is the currency of philanthropy. Gates correctly argued medical research and education, which was lacking in America at time, was the place for the most impact given the medical landscape.

Gates was correct, medicine in America was ripe for innovation and investments to catch up to European countries. The Rockefeller Institute for Medical Research was born in 1901, now named Rockefeller University. It was modeled on the Pasteur Institute in France and the Koch Institute in Germany. It focused on basic medical research and biomedical engineering and eventually a clinical component was added to the center as well. The Rockefeller Institute produced twenty-five Nobel laureates and became a model for medical research.

The Rockefeller Institute was a turning point for America in medical research. Germany, which was the epicenter and the model of medical and basic science research, had found a competitor in the New World. The Institute by itself did not change the dynamics of research or the balance of power in medicine. But the confluence of certain political events vaulted America into the forefront of medical research and discovery. The tragic and confounding start of World War I, which was called the Great War back then, significantly degraded Germany's standing in Europe. Led by its monarchy but without a clear objective, Germany thrust itself into a war it was ill-prepared for. The inconclusive end to World War I and the unfair terms for Germany (as perceived by Germans) led to the rise of the Third Reich and the ensuing devastation of Germany and continental Europe during World War II. After World War II, the center of medical and scientific research and innovation was positively moved to America. By escaping the devastation of World War II, America became the leader in basic science research which it has retained over the past century.

One of Rockefeller's contemporaries was Andrew Carnegie (1835–1919) who was a Scottish immigrant with a similarly modest start. He started work at a young age at a cotton factory. He had various jobs but eventually became a superintendent at a Pennsylvanian railroad company. He made various investments in coal, iron, and the railroad and, in his early thirties, he became a wealthy man. He founded a steel company near Pittsburgh during the 1870s and became wealthy beyond his imagination. The company he created was eventually bought by John Pierpont Morgan in 1901 for $480 million.

During his career as an industrialist, Carnegie considered himself the champion of the working people. However, his actions were sometimes contrary to his stated intent as he was notorious for violently breaking up strikes, stifling competition, and negotiating low wages with his workers. Nonetheless, he wanted to be perceived as a man of the people. He wrote an essay titled the *Gospel of Wealth*. In it, he argued for the responsibilities that wealthy men of society should accept, including caring for the welfare of society and its people. He famously said, "The man who dies thus rich, dies disgraced." It is quite possible it was Carnegie's influence which prompted Rockefeller to start his endeavor in philanthropy. Carnegie genuinely believed in giving away his wealth for public welfare and followed through while alive. He gave away most, if not all, of his wealth away to build libraries and music halls in America and worldwide. He endowed many organizations which are still active today. One of those foundations, the Carnegie Foundation for the Advancement of

Teaching, was established in 1905 and funded grants for research in education.

Henry Pritchett (1857–1939), who was the president of Carnegie foundation, was seeking scholars to study American education. He was intrigued by a book published by a Kentuckian, criticizing American education. Abraham Flexner (1866–1959) published his book titled *The American College, A Criticism* in 1908. Pritchett liked his work and asked Flexner to report on ways to improve medical education in America. The only problem was that Abraham Flexner had never set foot in a medical school or a teaching hospital. He was born to German immigrants in Kentucky and was the first in his family to attend college. He received a degree from Johns Hopkins University in classical studies. He was an educator tasked with finding a solution for the American medical educational system.

Abraham Flexner published his work in 1910. The report was called the *Flexner Report,* or Carnegie Foundation Bulletin Number Four, and had a huge impact on medical education in America. He reviewed and visited more than 155 medical schools in the United States and Canada. Most of the medical schools were no more than trade schools taught by local physicians for profit. Some students were able to practice medicine after a mere two years of education. There were a few medical schools which were connected to major universities. His assessment of American medical education was harsh. He called certain medical schools a plague or a disgrace. He found that medical education was not structured or uniform throughout the country, producing very poorly trained physicians.

He found one university which he regarded as a bright spot and to be used as an example for other schools to follow. Not surprisingly, he recommended his alma mater, Johns Hopkins University, as a model for medical education. He recommended at least two years of university education before admission to medical school and two years of basic science education followed by two years of clinical education under full-time faculty devoted to charity care and education. According to Flexner, training of new physicians should be at least six years and preferably eight years long. He recommended state regulations for medical schools and medical licenses. Each state should have jurisdiction over their medical schools and should grant them accreditation in conjunction with the Council of Medical Education which was formed by American Medical Association in 1904.

His most drastic recommendation was to close those schools who were not part of universities or did not have high standards. He recommended reducing the number of medical schools to thirty-one from 155. His report had concluded that most of those schools were profit centers for the local doctors and did not produce any benefit to the population. Instead of reforming them, they should be closed permanently, he recommended. From the year the report was published in 1910 to 1920, the number of medical schools in the country went from almost 160 to barely eighty. By the 1930s, there were only sixty-six medical schools in the country graduating physicians and most were affiliated with a university.

The main effect of the Flexner Report was the reduction of medical school graduates. In 1910, some 4,400 medical students graduated from American medical schools. By 1920, there were only 3,000 medical school graduates. Some of the medical schools that were forced to shut their doors were training women and African

Americans. Only two medical schools training African Americans survived the purge. It was a setback for women and minority physicians in the field of medicine. The effects lasted many decades until a conscientious effort was made to admit women and minorities to medical schools.

The reduction of medical school entrants made the selection criteria more stringent and the educational reform produced better-trained physicians. In turn, the prestige of medical graduates in America increased along with their paychecks. The states strictly regulated medical schools and the practice of medicine. The freewheeling, entrepreneurial, "market-based" nature of medical practice ceased to exist. The standard of care and the quality of physicians also increased, and the public was ultimately served well. The so-called "quacks," the alternative physicians in other fields besides approved MD schools, were put out of business. Medical education and the practice of medicine in America became uniform, homogenous, and high quality. Flexner's blueprint for medical education and the licensure of the practice of medicine is still enforced and followed more than one hundred years later.

While Abraham Flexner reformed medical education in America, his brother Simon Flexner (1863–1946), who was a physician with a degree from Johns Hopkins University, became the first director of the Rockefeller Institute. Simon Flexner was an accomplished researcher who was instrumental in emulating the German model of laboratory science. He was a successful director of the institute from 1901 to 1935. He advanced America's basic science research, while Abraham reformed medical education by incorporating basic science research and teaching as part of medical education. The two brothers, more than any other individuals, made a great impact on medicine in America and laid the foundation for a century of American dominance in medical discovery and education.

The two tycoons, Rockefeller and Carnegie, and the Flexner brothers truly revolutionized the education and practice of medicine in America. These two rich tycoons' philanthropic endeavors were, however, inspired by what transpired some twenty-five years earlier.

In the 1870s, another wealthy businessman by the name of Johns Hopkins (1795–1873) donated $7 million to the creation of a hospital and a university in the city of Baltimore. Johns Hopkins, who worked in his parents' plantation in Maryland as a young boy, worked his way up in retail and invested in railroad companies to become a wealthy man. He was a Quaker who witnessed his parents emancipating their slaves in 1807 which left a great impression on him. He was an abolitionist before Abraham Lincoln rose to presidency.

His philanthropic activities and charity preceded Carnegie's *Gospel of Wealth* by twenty-five years. Johns Hopkins witnessed multiple cholera outbreaks in Baltimore and those events prompted him to reduce suffering by establishing a hospital and a medical university. Daniel Coit Gilman (1831–1908) became the first president of Johns Hopkins University and he modeled it based on the German graduate education system. He integrated research and teaching which became the blueprint for the Flexner brothers, who both received their degrees from Johns Hopkins University.

Johns Hopkins University eventually established a nursing school, a public health school, and a publishing press. It became the model for all the institutions in America. Johns Hopkins University is still the preeminent place for medical education and research. Johns

Hopkins was a childless bachelor who accumulated wealth during his business career. His accumulated wealth did not go to waste but spawned an endeavor which has benefited mankind for more than a century. The donation of $7 million that Johns Hopkins gave to the school upon his death was the biggest donation to a university up to that point. He truly revolutionized medicine with his act of generosity and his legacy lives on after 140 years. Johns Hopkins University became the leading medical institution worldwide and a model for excellence to be emulated and, by proxy, Johns Hopkins became the model for philanthropy and legacy building. After Johns Hopkins, wealthy men looked to health issues and causes to create immortal legacies.

At the turn of the 21st century, America was the leading center for medical discovery and education. Hopkins, Rockefeller, Carnegie, Gilman, and the Flexner brothers created the foundation of medical education, research, and practice, which has lasted more than a century and has benefited millions.

Chapter 10

From Barber to Surgeon

Hippocrates, who is considered the father of medicine by many people around the globe, established the precedence for a knowledgeable and respectable physician. He considered a true physician to be the one who treats patients medically. Since surgery had a high rate of infection and the outcomes were not satisfactory in those early days, Hippocrates discouraged his students from engaging in the surgical treatments of patients. Hippocrates' motto of "first do no harm" was not consistent with the practice of surgery in those days. Patients usually ended up worse with those procedures. From Hippocrates' time, the people who practiced surgery on patients were considered part of a less prestigious profession and were not held in high regard by Hippocrates and his disciples.

This stigma of the surgical profession lasted many centuries. Initially, the people who practiced surgery were called barbers, not physicians. The practice of surgery was a gruesome affair. The barber did not practice antiseptic techniques, anesthesia was nonexistent, and the outcomes for the patients were horrific. The surgeries performed were mainly on superficial organs. A barber's daily job was lancing boils, treating fractures, sewing wounds, bloodletting, and removing skin growths. The only operation which was daring was the extraction of bladder stones. The operation was first described by

Celsus in the 1st century. It was advanced by Mariano Santo di Barletta (1488–1550). The stone was extracted from the bladder through the urethra which usually caused massive bleeding and incontinence. The practice of surgery was not where the early pioneers of medicine spent their time and efforts. Surgery, which derives from the Latin word *chirurgia* (meaning work of hands), was considered manual labor and a true physician was a thinker-philosopher, not a butcher. Therefore, surgery was considered an inferior (very inferior) subclass of medicine if it was even considered a part of medicine at all.

The first, great surgeon to greatly enhance the reputation of surgery in the field of medicine was the French surgeon Guy de Chauliac (1298–1368). He was the physician of Pope Clement VI and Pope Innocent VI. After studying medicine in Montpellier, the epicenter of medical education in France, he went to study anatomy under Nicola Bertuccio. There, he developed and mastered the art of surgery. He became famous and gained recognition during the Black Death when many physicians refused to treat patients and fled big cities. He survived the plague and his service to the public did not go unnoticed by the papacy. His greatest contribution was his book on surgery, *Chirurgia Magna*, which was probably the first book wholly on the subject of surgery. *Chirurgia Magna* was published in the 14th century which included many references to Galen, Avicenna, and Razi. His great work was distorted during the Reformation and Renaissance when most references to Islamic physicians were removed from many medical textbooks including Chauliac's great work.

By the Middle Ages, the practice of surgery still had not changed much. The medical profession was divided into three classes. The physicians were the unquestioned leaders of the medical world and set the standard in practice of medicine. The surgeons were the second class of doctors who treated patients with procedures which had not changed much over the centuries. There was animosity between those two groups of healers, but society had a higher regard for the physician than the surgeon. What united physicians and surgeons was their disdain for the "ignorant" barbers. In the Middle Ages, the rivalry and turf battles among physicians, surgeons, and barbers was intense. Most surgeons were educated through apprenticeships as opposed to formal medical education which most physicians received. Knowing their status in the hierarchy of medicine, surgeons began to organize to enhance their position within the hierarchy of medicine. In the 13th century, surgeons formed guilds which provided training for aspiring surgeons. The trainees started wearing short robes and once they received adequate training to become surgeons and perform surgery on patients, they would wear long robes signifying proficiency in surgery. There were scholars who claimed that barber-surgeons wore short robes and physicians wore long robes to differentiate between the two professions. Regardless of who wore which size robes, the short robes were inferior and so were the barber-surgeons.

Eventually barbers joined surgeons to form a united front in their battle against physicians. In England, it took an act of parliament to form a barber-surgeon company which merged the two professions together. After the 16th century, most barbers merged with surgeons and the field of surgery was solidified in the practice of medicine. The politicking of the surgical practice was settled in the 16th century, but the profession still lacked any appreciative breakthroughs. After the merger of barbers and surgeons, the surgical outcomes and structured training were still horrible. The field of surgery was successful in organizing and solidifying their position but lacked visionaries or capable innovators to bring respectability to the profession. In 1745, surgeons separated from barbers to form their own guild and, to this day, surgeons are still called "Mister" and not "Doctor" in England.

During the Renaissance, Ambroise Paré (1510–1590) was probably the best-known surgeon. He trained to be a barber-surgeon at the oldest hospital in Paris, Hotel-Dieu. Like many surgeons before him and since, he perfected his craft attending to wounded soldiers. The wars during those periods were gruesome and the injuries devastating. Battlefield medicine became a full-time profession for some barber-surgeons. Paré experimented with treating wounds differently and with different substances. Some he treated with hot oil and some he treated with an ointment consisting of egg yolk, roses, and turpentine. He realized the wounds treated by the ointment fared better and healed faster than the ones treated by hot oil. He realized that cauterization, using heat to stop the bleeding, was very painful and ligature of the arteries worked better and was less painful for the patients. His first book, *The Method of Curing Wounds Caused by Arquebus and Firearms*, was instrumental in helping other barber-surgeons working in battlefields. He eventually became barber-surgeon to multiple kings in France until his death at the age of eighty. It is worth noting that, in his spare time when he was a young barber-surgeon, he gave people shaves and haircuts before he became a renowned battlefield surgeon.

The origin of barbers performing surgery probably started when the papacy forbade the clergy from shedding blood in 1163. The monks were required to have regular bloodletting and their peers usually performed the procedure. Since the church forbade the practice and they were required to have regular bloodletting, they turned to barbers to perform the procedure. The barbers were part of most monasteries since the 10th and 11th centuries because the clergy had to be clean shaven. The physicians did not protest the decision to let barbers perform bloodletting because most physicians regarded the act of performing surgery beneath their dignity and were happy to let someone else perform it. It was also the case that most surgical procedures did not have good outcomes and the physicians were happy to let someone else take the fall for the botched surgeries which was usually the case. Physicians maintained their lofty position and outsourced the act of surgery with its usually bad outcomes to barbers who were happy to accept a new source of income. Most barber-surgeons did perform shaves and haircuts until they were officially separated in the 18th century into two different fields.

Like many professions, surgery needed an event to break out of its inferior role and become prominent. The daily work of a barber-surgeon was very mundane and not rewarding. It was lancing boils, and bloodletting, usually at the request of a patient, or grisly amputations without anesthesia or antisepsis. Surgery's time to shine arrived courtesy of His Royal Anus, Louis the XIV. The Sun King, as he was known, was a very powerful and consequential ruler of France. In 1687, His Royal Highness developed a swelling in his anal region. The king's physician kept an eye on the swelling (that's what physicians did those days, watched it) but the swelling and pain only increased. The king developed an abscess and eventually a fistula developed. The Sun King could not ride his horse or sit on his throne (literally). The court physicians watched the fistula for a long period of time and realized that the king's condition was not getting any better. The fistula was interfering with the king's daily responsibilities.

The royal physicians sought a barber-surgeon to perform a procedure to heal the king's anus since the physicians did not know how to do it and had never done any cutting on people. They sought the help of a local Parisian barber-surgeon, Charles-Francois Félix (1650–1703). Realizing the enormity of the task—he would be cutting open the king after all—Félix wisely didn't proceed with surgery immediately. He astutely recruited patients from the poor section of town and the local prison to perform the surgery and practice the operation before performing it on the king. After months of performing the surgery sometimes on otherwise healthy patients, he developed certain instruments to perform the surgery.

After months of practice on poor patients, he performed the surgery on the royal fistula. The surgery was a success. The king was able to sit and, after a few months, he was able to ride his horse and the recovery was a smashing success. The barber-surgeon's moment had arrived and was seized by Félix, changing the reputation of the field. Surgery ceased to be inferior to physicians and started to ascend in the hierarchy of medical practice. Félix was handsomely rewarded by the Sun King. He was given money, title, and land. Louis XV, Louis XIV's grandson, opened the Royal Academy of Surgery in 1731. Surgery became a part of medical teaching along with other disciplines and surgery merged with medical education rather than be a separate field inferior to physicians. The royal ass did more for the discipline of surgery than any other event or person. In short, the royal bum changed the face of surgery.

Once surgery became a part of medical education, its fortune and profile rose. During the 18th century, surgery benefited greatly as part of medical education. The 19th century was surgery's breakout century. During this period, surgeons performed in big theaters in many great medical schools. The surgeons were like performers entering the ring, with spectators all around watching in awe at the spectacle of blood, scalpel, pain, and suffering in the spirit of healing the patient. The surgeon's prowess and excellence were his speed. Since there was no anesthesia, the faster the surgeon performed his surgery, the less time the patient suffered the excruciating pain. It was said that the brilliance of surgery was measured by a stopwatch. To save time, some surgeons held the knife in their mouths during the surgery to shorten the procedure time. Surgeons moved to the forefront of medicine with the array of surgeries they were performing. Some surgeries were unsuccessful or unsupported by evidence but still became widely utilized such as tongue surgery for stuttering.

Most surgeries during the 19th century were still on superficial organs. No one had dared to open up someone's belly to cut an organ out. The most daring surgery which was commonly performed was amputations. The next breakthrough in surgery came from the United States. In Europe, the field of medicine and surgery was tightly controlled with several regulations to prevent abuse. The great universities of Europe admonished surgeons who became too daring and the professional guilds would expel surgeons if their practice was deemed unsafe. In America, the practice of medicine was poorly, if at all, regulated. Physicians had more leeway to experiment and perform cutting-edge treatments without any repercussions.

As expected, the first pioneering surgery on a patient was performed in America when Jane Todd Crawford presented to Ephraim McDowell (1771–1830) with an abdominal mass. Ms. Crawford's physician first suspected a pregnancy but later realized that it was a mass inside her stomach and not a baby. He referred her to Dr. McDowell who practiced in Danville, Kentucky. McDowell explained the risk of removing the tumor and the pioneering nature of the procedure since it had never been attempted before. Ms. Crawford accepted all the risks and traveled to McDowell's house for the surgery. The surgery took twenty-five minutes without anesthesia. She sang songs to drown out the pain. McDowell was able to remove the ovarian tumor from her abdomen and she recovered and lived for another thirty-two years. It proved that abdominal surgery was possible and opened the door for more daring surgeries.

Another American surgeon who pioneered gynecological surgery was James Marion Sims (1813–1883). He was able to examine patients with vesico-vaginal fistulas—essentially ruptures in the wall separating the bladder from the vagina—utilizing a new speculum he had devised. Sims practiced in Alabama and had many slave patients with vesico-vaginal fistulas which can occur after labor. He experimented by employing different approaches to repair vaginal tears and fistulas. He was able to successfully repair some of the fistulas and traveled to New York to establish a hospital for women. He traveled to Europe to demonstrate his novel approach and the surgical procedure became prevalent in America and Europe.

The field of gynecology took shape before the use of anesthesia. Women were subjected to many gynecological procedures which were not safe or effective in hopes of finding the next breakthrough procedure. Women, and especially slave women, suffered a lot during those early days of pioneering surgery. It is reported that Sims operated on a slave thirty-three times to correct a fistula. The abuse and malpractice in gynecological surgery was prevalent even in Europe where medicine was more regulated. Isaac Baker Brown (1812–1873) became a specialist in clitoridectomies in London. The husbands would bring their wives whom they deemed nymphomaniacs to have the procedure done to them. The practice was so lucrative that it attracted the attention of the local obstetric society. Brown was expelled from the society, not because of the practice, but because of self-promotion and not obtaining proper consent. Brown moved to America to continue his practice because of lax regulations. Women were part of the pioneering work of many surgeons in the 19th century and the abuse they received should never be brushed under the rug. Many surgeons participated in the practice with few voices airing concerns until Elizabeth Blackwell, the first woman to graduate from medical school.

Even after those pioneering intra-abdominal surgeries performed by American surgeons, there were many limitations to surgery. Two main obstacles for surgeons and patients to undertake surgery was pain and infection. Most patients preferred to die than undergo the knife because of the amount of pain and uneven outcomes. There were multiple forms of pain management during surgery in those days. Opium, which was used extensively in the Middle East, was one mode of pain control and alcohol was another. These substances did not sufficiently alleviate the pain of amputations and other new, daring procedures.

The first reported use of gases to induce euphoria was reported in 1800 by Humphry Davy (1778–1829). He reported that inhaling nitrous oxide produced giggling and dizziness. He claimed that inhaling the gas mixed with oxygen could also alleviate pain and could be used for surgery. No one noticed his report or made use of the groundbreaking experiment.

Another gas, ether, was also finding a market, especially in American fairs. It was dubbed "laughing gas." People who tried the gas at fairs and parties would giggle and fall to the ground drunk. Witnessing these parties, William E. Clarke, a physician from New York, extracted a tooth under ether in 1842. The operation was a success. A few months later, another surgeon in Georgia, Crawford Long (1815–1878), witnessed that, when people inhaled the gas, they did not feel any pain upon falling to the ground. Apparently, Dr. Long himself had participated in those laughing gas parties so he had firsthand knowledge. He administered ether to James Venable during the removal of a cyst from his neck. The surgery was a success and the patient recovered well.

Ether became mainstream when Horace Wells (1815–1848), a dentist in the New England area, was so impressed by ether that he had one of his own teeth extracted under ether anesthesia in 1844. He was so convinced of the effects and its usefulness in surgery that he made an apparatus to administer the gas. He convinced John Collins Warren (1778–1856) to try the gas during his lectures to extract a tooth from a patient. The live demonstration was a disaster.

The patient experienced tremendous pain during the procedure and the whole experiment was a total catastrophe.

Ether would get a second chance with William Thomas Green Morton (1819–1868), a Boston dentist, convinced Dr. Warren to try his machine for surgery. Morton had done experiments on dogs, himself, and a patient and was more comfortable using gas. He practiced the art of anesthesia before convincing the same Dr. Warren to try it on a patient. On October 16th, 1846, Dr. Warren successfully removed a tumor from the neck of patient at Massachusetts General Hospital under anesthesia administered by Morton. The surgery was a smashing success and the proper administration of ether during surgery became accepted. Soon, the new discovery spread to many parts of Europe and surgeons were using ether for anesthesia. A new dawn in surgery was upon mankind. Anesthesia conquered the pain patients felt during surgery and painful surgery became a thing of the past. Patients slept through procedures with that wonderful gas.

Another chemical also became popular for surgery. Chloroform, which was initially used by James Young Simpson (1811–1870) in the mid-1800s, displaced ether in some European countries. Simpson, who was a faculty of surgery member in Edinburgh, was successful in promoting chloroform which was easier to administer and did not cause the vomiting associated with ether. Chloroform got its break when Queen Victoria received chloroform during delivery in 1853. If it was good enough for the queen, it sure was good enough for the masses.

Ether- and chloroform-induced general anesthesia was not entirely safe in those early days. The next big break to lessen the pain of surgery came from Sigmund Freud (1856–1939). He was not a surgeon but had friends in the field of surgery. In discussions with his friend and colleague Carl Koller (1857–1944), Freud mentioned that cocaine, which was used to treat some psychiatric disorders (and Freud was known to use it), numbed the tongue after tasting it. Intrigued by the numbing properties of cocaine, Dr. Koller used it during surgery to numb the eye and the patient did not experience much pain. Cocaine became the first local anesthetic and later Merck started mass producing cocaine for local anesthesia. Eventually, lidocaine, a synthetic substance, replaced cocaine. Cocaine was still used up until the 1990s for some eye surgeries. General anesthesia and local anesthesia transformed the art and science of surgery. Surgery was ascendant after the triumph over surgical pain.

Pain was conquered by ether and local anesthesia, but infections still hindered many patients seeking surgical treatments. There were many competing arguments for the reason of high infection rates in those days. Through small incremental steps, the rate of infections was reduced, and a few clinicians deserve the credit for making surgery safer for patients. The first breakthrough came in Vienna. Ignaz Semmelweis (1818–1865) was a physician in Vienna General Hospital where many women went for childbirth. There were two maternity wards, one manned by medical students and the other by midwives. The postpartum infection rates were much higher in the ward which was attended by medical students while the other ward had a lower infection rate. He switched the staff of the two wards and, to his surprise, the high infection rate followed the medical students to the new ward. He was convinced that the infection rate was caused by the behavior of the medical students and that it was preventable since the midwives had a much smaller infection rate. Looking for the cause, he caught a break with a tragic event. Jakob Kolletschka (1803–1847), a physician Semmelweis knew, accidentally cut his finger while performing an autopsy and later died of an infection. He died of the same infection as the dead body. Semmelweis concluded that the infection was carried by the medical students from the autopsy area to the maternity ward. Medical students would attend autopsies and would take their instruments from the morgue to the maternity ward, spreading infections.

In 1847, he ordered handwashing with chlorinated water before tending to patients and deliveries. The results were miraculous. The rate of postpartum infections plummeted, and he was convinced in the communicable nature of the infections. Most physicians were not convinced and challenged his findings and recommendations. He quit his post and moved to Budapest and was eventually admitted to a psychiatric hospital. Time and new science vindicated his recommendations and handwashing became and still is the cornerstone of preventing infections.

Surgery in the mid-19th century was still a messy affair. Surgeons would walk into operating rooms with their street clothes and start performing surgeries on patients. There were spectators and anyone interested could walk in and watch. Great surgeons would perform their surgeries in theaters like in the old Roman coliseum. This environment was not conducive to sterile surgery. Anesthesia had conquered pain but the post-operative course for many patients was still perilous. Most patients would develop severe infections with a high rate of mortality.

Surgeons started paying attention to the high infection and mortality rates after surgery and there was a debate as to the cause of these infections. Pasteur and Koch had demonstrated that bacteria caused infections. With his experiments, Pasteur revealed that bacteria existed in the air and could cause infections. An English surgeon, Joseph Lister (1827–1912), concerned about high rate of infections set out to reduce the incidence. He read Louis Pasteur research and was impressed by germ theory. Pasteur's conclusion regarding the elimination of microorganisms included heat, filtration, and chemical exposure. It was not feasible to apply heat to the patient's open wound or use filtration for surgical purposes. However, chemical exposure could be useful in elimination of microorganism and could be applied to a patient's wound.

He discovered that carbolic acid was used to treat sewage and the same field which was treated with carbolic acid was safe for grazing by livestock. He initially applied carbolic acid to a young boy's fracture wound and the patient's wound and fracture healed well without any sequelae. He proceeded to apply the carbolic acid to the patients' wounds, soaked the surgical instruments in carbolic acid, and sprayed it around the operating room. His infection rate plummeted after using carbolic acid as a prevention of infection. The success of his aseptic technique was unquestionably remarkable. In 1867, Listor published his results and experience with carbolic acid in *Lancet* and soon his aseptic practice was copied in many countries around Europe and eventually in America. Like many pioneers before him, his ideas and aseptic practice were initially mocked. Eventually, his idea of aseptic surgical standard was proven by the new laboratory science blossoming in the late 19th century. He deserved a lot of the credit for introducing and moving surgery to a safer plateau. With his technique, it became possible to perform more daring surgeries inside many of body's cavities which was never attempted before. Brain, abdominal, and chest surgeries were now a possibility with low infection rates and soon surgeons pushed the boundaries of traditional operations.

Other aseptic techniques found their way into operating rooms. American surgeon William Halsted (1852–1922) introduced rubber gloves to the practice of medicine. Incidentally, his creation was meant for a different purpose. Dr. Halsted's nurse and fiancé complained of hand dermatitis from using the chemicals during the sterilization of instruments. He had Goodyear make thin, rubber gloves to prevent irritation of a provider's skin. It eventually was shown the benefit to the patient and ability to aid in preventing infection. The discovery of droplet infections led to the use of surgical masks and eventually surgical gowns. The operating rooms became isolated rooms in hospitals with restricted entry and strict dress codes which included masks, gloves, and gowns as well as sterile instruments. Researchers, including Koch, found that heat was superior to chemicals in sterilizing instruments and heating became the standard sterilization technique.

Surgery, just like laboratory work, entered the microscopic stage. The first use of a microscope on a live person was when ophthalmologists used a binocular microscope to look at the cornea in 1899. The first reported case of a microscopic surgery was performed by an ear specialist in the early 20th century. The 20th-century surgeons, armed with anesthesia, aseptic techniques, microscopes, and antibiotics pushed the limits of what was possible in surgery which was unimaginable at the turn of the century. By the end of the 20th century, surgeons were operating on fetuses inside women's uteruses.

Barbers morphed into barber-surgeons, forced their way into medical universities, and became part of medical education. Shedding the barber part of their profession, they made strides in making surgery safer and, with the diminishing risks, leaped to the top of the medical hierarchy with high rewards and prestige. The act of surgery may have been akin to butchery in the Middle Ages, but it transformed into the sleek profession of people with good hands and confidence to do what was almost impossible a century earlier. First considered indignant work, the field of surgery became the cornerstone of many reputable hospitals and universities and continues to create exceptional results for patients to this day.

Chapter 11

Wars and The Great Leap of Medicine

Humans organized themselves into small communities and civilization took hold in Mesopotamia thousands of years ago. There were many benefits to living close together. They were able to help each other in daily activities, food could be harvested in efficient ways, and individuals with expertise in certain areas could provide a service to community members. With close associations with each other, however, one main drawback soon became evident. People, by nature, are protective of their belongings and their immediate property. When people were drawn to live close to each other, there was a higher incidence of conflict among members. The proximity of people caused increased interactions, misunderstandings, and eventually hostilities.

When rival towns were formed in close proximity to each other, the same tendency to resort to conflict became apparent. The closeness of people, towns, and civilizations inevitably led to major conflicts and wars. Some of the bloodiest wars in history occurred in the Middle East and Europe, two places with many different cultures and concentrated in small areas. Historically, the two bloodiest wars are World War II, where Europe ripped itself apart, and the Mongolian Invasion of Persia, where the Middle East was ripped apart. Wars have been part of human history since civilizations formed, and societies could organize a standing army to combat each other. As human societies advanced from villages to countries and empires the wars became deadlier and more brutal.

There is no doubt that wars leave a lasting scar on the losers and victors alike. Though it's difficult to consider, the more brutal the war, the more opportunity there was for the science of medicine and surgery to advance. Some of the best surgeons received their training during those brutal wars. Galen got his start repairing men who fought each other as gladiators. Ambroise Paré, the great French barber-surgeon, perfected his surgical skills as a battlefield surgeon during the campaign of Francis I. As many physicians believed, if one wanted to be a great surgeon, he should go to war zones. The wars throughout history have been ruthless. Before guns, battlefield injuries were mutilations with hammers, axes, and swords and provided field surgeons ample opportunity to practice surgery without any repercussions. Wounded soldiers provided plenty of cases for surgeons to experiment and advance the art of surgery.

Surgeons were not the only benefactors of the wars that humans have fought. Probably a shining development of any war came during the Crimean War in the 1850s. The British Empire was involved in a regional war against Russia. The ruthlessness of the war produced many casualties for the British army. Unsanitary conditions and a lack of supplies resulted in many deaths of British soldiers and sailors. Appalled by the treatment of soldiers, there was public outrage regarding the treatment of the war wounded. The Crimean War produced a genuine heroine in a woman named Florence Nightingale (1820–1910).

Nightingale was born to a wealthy British family in Florence, Italy. She was raised in a home where she was expected to behave like ladies of upper-class society in England. She had many clashes with her mother because she did not conform to her mother's standards and expectations. She was educated in classic English fashion, learning languages, the arts, and mathematics. Despite growing up in the family mansion, she was always interested in the poor and ill people who lived close to their home. She would tend to them and take care of the sick, poor people of the area. Realizing her joy and passion to help others, she approached her parents for permission to attend nursing school. In 19th century Europe, women did not attend medical school and it was not a possibility for any woman including Florence. Her parents suggested marrying a gentleman from the same upper-class society. She refused the marriage proposal and enrolled at the Institution of Protestant Deaconesses in Germany.

Nursing education was mostly at religious institutions. Religious institutions were active in caring for the poor and sick and most hospitals had some affiliations with churches where most nurses came from. For centuries, nuns cared for the sick and the poor and doing the same at a hospital was no different than caring for the poor on the streets. After graduating from nursing school, Nightingale returned to London and became well-known for her promptness and the cleanliness of the wards where she was in charge. Her managerial skills impressed many on Harley Street where the leading figures of medicine practiced in London.

In 1854, the British War Secretary tasked Florence Nightingale with organizing a relief effort to tend to the wounded in

Constantinople. She organized a team of nurses and sailed to Crimea. When they arrived at Scutari, the military hospital, they were shocked to find the hospital in such filthy condition. Patients were lying in their own feces on stretchers in hallways. There were bugs and rats roaming the hospital corridors with no supplies or help. She set in motion a plan of action to clean the hospital from floor to ceiling. She tasked able-bodied patients with cleaning their area. Laundry service was started so patients could have clean linens. A kitchen was established to provide warm and nutritious meals and a library for intellectual stimulation for the patients and staff. She worked tirelessly to transform a filthy building into what became a model for future hospitals.

She would go around at night with a lamp in her hand making rounds to make sure all the patients were comfortable and attended to. She was dubbed the "Lady with the Lamp" who brought comfort. Others named her the Angel of Crimea. In 1856 at the conclusion of the war, she returned home to a hero's welcome. Queen Victoria rewarded her with an engraved brooch which became known as Nightingale Jewel. She established a hospital and nursing school for future students and brought respectability and professionalism to the field of nursing. The field of nursing was transformed by her actions, determination, and perseverance. Nursing became a noble profession and was no longer frowned upon by upper-class members.

Some of the giants of medicine served in wars where they gained invaluable experience. Robert Koch, Pasteur's competitor and the great German microbiologist, served as an army surgeon during the Franco-Prussian War. His work on anthrax began on battlefields observing the nature of the infections and the dormancy period of the *Bacillus anthracis*. In the same Franco-Prussian War, the French surgeon amputated more than 10,000 limbs with a sepsis rate exceeding 75%. This tragic mortality rate was the impetus to pay attention to Listor and adopt his aseptic techniques.

Alexander Fleming served during World War I and he observed the tetanus epidemic among soldiers and the treatment which was effective. He was encouraged that infections could be defeated and discovered penicillin. When penicillin was ultimately mass produced in America, it was first used during World War II. Allied soldiers in North Africa were treated with penicillin which was a new drug. Thankfully for the soldiers, penicillin worked, but the soldiers and their horrific wounds provided the human experimental subjects to test a new drug and gauge its effectiveness.

World War I was the first devasting war staged on a global scale. The weapons used during the Great War, as it was called, were new and more powerful than any previous war. There were tanks, explosives, powerful guns, and bombs that ripped people open. The wounds soldiers suffered during World War I were never seen on the battlefield before. Just like societies in that era were going through a transition in transportation, wars were also in transition to the modern era. On the battlefields, horses were still used, and horse manure was present on most battlefields causing severe infection and providing an opportunity for physicians to treat unusual infections. The massive wounds soldiers suffered were exposed to much of the dirty environment around them. Tetanus, which is common in soil and horse manure, caused an epidemic among the soldiers. The Allies and Germans had major outbreaks of tetanus during the war. Tetanus, which is caused by *Clostridium tetani*, causes muscle spasms, nervous system dysfunction, high blood pressure, among many other symptoms, and became an issue for the wounded soldiers.

A scientist from Koch's institute had discovered a horse serum to combat diphtheria and tetanus, but it was not widely used. Given the outbreak on the battlefield and the casualties it was causing to soldiers on both sides, anti-tetanus serum was mass produced and used on the battlefields. The necessary caution and trials before mass use of antitoxins were discarded for the sake of expediency. The army had to look for a solution and implement it fast since defeat and victory were at stake.

Soldiers on both sides of the battle received the antitoxin and thousands died of the reaction it caused. Most, however, survived the treatment and the tetanus outbreak was successfully controlled. The soldiers were yet again the necessary test subjects for medicine to experiment and perfect its treatments and remedies. A lot was learned during those outbreaks and the solutions were later studied further, but the rapid implementation and analysis of the treatment could not have been done during peacetime. The Great War ended in a stalemate and the inconclusive resolution to the war led to another more catastrophic war than the Great War, World War II.

World War II was more devastating than the first and is widely considered the deadliest war in human history. It ripped a continent apart. The wealth of many nations was squandered in pursuit of fascism and totalitarianism. Brutal wars were instrumental in the advancement of the field of surgery. As discussed in the previous chapter, surgery had gone through a metamorphosis and changed drastically in a hundred years, more so than it had in preceding 2,000 years. Anesthesia, aseptic techniques, and antibiotics made many, previously unthinkably surgeries possible. Orthopedic surgery and plastic surgery made great advances repairing maimed soldiers. After World War II started in 1939, just twenty years after World War I, the lessons learned during the first war were still fresh in most surgeons' minds and were applied in the new war zones. They built on the experience during the first war to perfect the art of battlefield medicine.

Every war produced an opportunity for medicine to advance. The Iran-Iraq war produced many soldiers who were exposed to chemical weapons used by Saddam Hussein. Medical literature is full of studies on those patients especially those who suffered corneal injury and blindness as well as their successful treatments. During the last major war, the second Iraq War, traumatic brain injury was managed, and strides were made to increase survival rates after major brain injuries. Decompressive craniectomy was shown to be effective in patients with severe brain injuries during the war which significantly improved the survival rates of soldiers. Decompressive craniectomy involves the removal of part of the skull to alleviate the intracranial pressure, and it proved remarkably beneficial to patients as opposed to medical management of the condition.

As long as there have been conflicts and wars, physicians and nurses have been there to help the afflicted. Through the chaos and mayhem, physicians were able to treat soldiers and learn invaluable lessons which would not have been possible in peacetime. It is hard to convince people to try a new medicine or try a new procedure when there are other options and the circumstances are not so dire. During war, any help and care in the brutal, stench-filled trenches was a blessing for the soldiers. They were willing to accept and submit to a lot when in pain and possibly dying in the dirt in a place far from home and alone at a young age. Many soldiers not only defended their countries or advanced a cause—whether right or wrong—but they also greatly contributed to the voyage of medicine and its advancement. The results have benefited countless people afterward.

It is worth noting that medicine and physicians have not always channeled their efforts into helping mankind and relieve their suffering. Two incidents in the history of warfare deserve to be mentioned and deeply dissected to explain the dark side of medicine during wars. Medicine has not always produced people like Nightingale during the Crimean War, or Paré during Francis I's campaign, or Alexander Fleming during World War I, or Koch during the Franco-Prussian War.

One of the dark incidents of medicine happened during World War II. Japan, a rising power in the Far East, was engaged in the Sino-Japanese War. Eventually Japan joined Germany to form the Axis and declared war on the United States by bombing Pearl Harbor. For most Western readers, the atrocities of Japan were limited to the experience they had or the tales they have read about Pearl Harbor as President Franklin said, "A date which will live in infamy." Closer to Japan, atrocities occurred with the help of medical professionals that are truly shocking to read and shake people's consciousness.

In the aftermath of World War I, the European powers experienced the lethal effects of biological and chemical warfare and the devastating effects it had on their population and, in turn, signed the Geneva Protocol which banned the use of chemical and biological weapons. Imperial Japan decided that those weapons must be very effective and set out to develop biological weapons. The management of this project was assigned to Imperial Army Officer Shirō Ishii (1892–1959), the leading physician in the army and trained microbiologist. Dr. Ishii set out to develop a program through systemic design adhering to research principles with accuracy and reproducibility of the tests.

He was brutally efficient in setting up the program. An area in China was developed with hundreds of buildings with nearby open fields for experimentations. The program, and the location, was called Unit 731. Unit 731 was probably established in the mid-1930s and the program ended with the surrender of Japan to the United States.

For the next fifteen years, the atrocities which occurred in this camp under the supervision of Dr. Ishii and his medical colleagues were stains on the profession and humanity. They gathered prisoners from surrounding areas, mostly Chinese men, with some Russians as well. Women and children were at the camp as well but not in high numbers. The researchers set to test the effectiveness of biological agents such as cholera, anthrax, and the bubonic plague on human subjects. They exposed healthy prisoners to the disease and would then vivisect the infected prisoners to study the effects of the biological agents. Vivisection is the dissection of a living human without anesthesia. A vivid description was given in the New York Times in 1995 by an assistant at Unit 731:

> The fellow knew that it was over for him, and so he didn't struggle when they led him into the room and tied him down.

But when I picked up the scalpel, that's when he began screaming. I cut him open from the chest to the stomach, and he screamed terribly, and his face was all twisted in agony. He made this unimaginable sound, he was screaming so horribly. But then finally he stopped. This was all in a day's work for the surgeons, but it really left an impression on me because it was my first time.

Some of the participants in these studies were questioned as to why they did not provide anesthesia to patients before dissecting them. The response was as shocking as the experiments: They claimed that it would affect the body and the results would vary if another agent entered the body. They wanted to dissect and observe the inside of the body in its natural form.

They subjected humans to freezing conditions, so they could study the effective treatment for frostbite. They performed experimental surgery on patients to study novel approaches. They removed the patient's stomach and attached the esophagus to the intestine to see if the patient could survive. Prisoners and sometimes mothers and children would be put in pressure chambers or gas chambers to study the effects of gas or pressure on different age groups.

Prisoners would be tied up in the field and bombs would explode at different distances to study the effectiveness of bomb developments. New biological weapons were tested on nearby villages to gauge its effectiveness. Wells would be poisoned to see if a germ was lethal.

During the war with the United States, Unit 731 was in the final stages of a mission to send planes with anthrax or bubonic plague on Kamikaze missions to infect coastal cities of the United States such as San Diego or balloons filled with germs to land in the middle of American cities. Thankfully, their darkest visions never came to fruition because they surrendered to the United States.

Before surrender, the Japanese army demolished the prison camp and destroyed the evidence. They released the infected rodents to the surrounding areas in China and infected more people in subsequent years. However, they kept meticulous records of all their evil experiments with some effective treatments such as proper treatment of frostbite. When the American forces captured Shirō Ishii, they gave him and his colleagues immunity in exchange for the data they had collected during their years at the camp. Dr. Ishii died of throat cancer in 1959 at the age of sixty-seven as a free man. He never faced any disciplinary action or jail time. His colleagues at Unit 731 continued to have good careers and rose to prominent positions in the post-war era.

Another evil figure in the history of medicine worked and lived during the dark period where Nazism was on the march in Europe. Josef Mengele (1911–1979), the Nazi physician who was stationed at the Auschwitz concentration camp, experimented on people in the name of medicine. He majored in anthropology at college and was very interested in and did studies on genetics while studying medicine. During the rise of Nazism in Germany, the leadership was obsessed with master race arguments. They considered the Aryan race to be superior to others and wanted to expand their homeland for the proliferation of the Aryan race. Mengele was interested in increasing the reproduction capabilities of the Aryan race through twin pregnancies and studied the genetic variation and effects of disease.

At Auschwitz, the selectors would choose people who were able to perform duties and those that were not able were sent to gas chambers. Mengele was involved in the selection process and would pick twins, mostly children, for his experiments. Heterochromia, people with different colored irises, were selected and killed and their eyes would be sent to a laboratory in Berlin for further study. He experimented on pregnant prisoners to study reproduction. Twins were subjected to different diseases and, if one was infected with a disease, he would kill both and send the bodies for comparative autopsies.

The extent of his evil experimentations was not fully exposed because he fled the camp with the camp's documents. He eventually fled to South America and lived there till his death. He was never brought to justice and his actions were not fully discovered. Most of the Nazi collaborators at those concentration camps fled or were killed and never shared their activities with invading armies, so a full account of what they did never materialized.

During wars, when a nation's existence is at stake, physicians are known to cross the line for the "good of the country." What Mengele and Ishii did are beyond the pale. The systemic cruelty they demonstrated to advance medical knowledge was never done before and should never be undertaken no matter what the cause. Even tinkering with practice standards during wars should not be allowed or condoned. Physicians should not participate in carrying out capital punishment or advise on ways to extract information under duress from prisoners. There is no justification for any activity which violates the patient-doctor relationship as described by Hippocrates and intentionally hurt the person under a physician's immediate care in hopes of helping others. Physicians should stand up to what's wrong in societies, not merely condone and assimilate the prevailing societal norms into the practice of medicine. The practice of medicine should be stalwart in opposing any actions which are contrary to the duty of caring and healing others in any society and under whatever system of governance.

Wars are never-ending nightmares for any soul unfortunate enough to experience it. This author experienced war as a child and would never wish such calamity on anyone. Wars have been around as long as man and will continue to happen. It is just human nature. Humanity occasionally takes a pause from conflict and inevitably the ugly events recur just as the morning sun appears every day. The physicians should be ready to alleviate the suffering and bring a sense of humanity and compassion to even the most dreadful of circumstances. We can only hope that the experience of helping others in war zones will help mankind later. One should not lose his moral bearing in pursuit of higher "honors." There is no higher honor than being entrusted with the duty of doing what's best for the person looking at you, asking for help.

Chapter 12

Medicine and Statesmen

"Medicine is a social science, and politics is nothing else but medicine on a large scale."
—Rudolf Virchow

When civilization was taking shape in Mesopotamia, some form of primitive healing was part of the fabric of that civilization. The healers were probably mostly local priests or magicians or sorcerers who tended to the sick. There was no code of conduct or science guiding their behavior or decisions. The interaction was between the patient and the healer in any form which suited the patient. The laws governing the interaction were solely at the discretion of the healer and the patient.

The first documented involvement of the state in medicine dates back to the 18th century BC. In Mesopotamia, a dynasty was taking shape in the 1500s BC. The Babylonian Dynasty produced many kings. One notable king was the sixth king of the dynasty: Hammurabi who reigned for forty-two years between 1792 BC to 1750 BC. He expanded the frontier of his reign to eventually control all of Mesopotamia in modern-day Iraq. In the thirtieth year of his rule, he produced a set of codes of conduct. His codes had 282 rules for the people of his kingdom. This is the first known documented legal code which was discovered in Susa, Iran, in 1901 and is currently displayed at the Louvre museum in Paris.

The legal code came to be known as the Code of Hammurabi. The codes are mostly about family laws, punishment for bad conduct such as stealing of property. Among the 282 codes, nine codes focused on the practice of medicine and two focused on veterinary medicine. The codes set fee schedules for medical services and appropriate punishments for cases of malpractice.

215. If a physician makes a large incision with an operating knife and cures it, or if he opens a tumor (over the eye) with an operating knife and saves the eye, he shall receive ten shekels.
216. If the patient is a freed man, he receives five shekels.
217. If he is the slave of someone, his owner shall give the physician two shekels.
218. If a physician makes a large incision with the operating knife and kills him, or opens a tumor with the operating knife and cuts out the eye, his hands shall be cut off.
219. If a physician makes a large incision in the slave of a freed man and kills him, he shall replace the slave with another slave.
220. If a physician opens a tumor with the operating knife and puts out his eye, he shall pay half his value.
221. If a physician heals the broken bone or diseased soft part of a man, the patient shall pay the physician five shekels.
222. If he is a freed man, he shall pay three shekels.

223. If he is a slave his owner shall pay the physician two shekels.
224. If a veterinary surgeon performs a serious operation on an ass or an ox and cures it, the owner shall pay the surgeon one-sixth of a shekel as a fee.
225. If he performs a serious operation on an ass or ox and kills it, he shall pay the owner one-fourth of its value.

As is evident, medicine and the practice of medicine were important parts of early civilizations and the conduct of physicians was a concern to ruling kings because they realized matters important to their subjects should be properly regulated and a code of conduct strictly enforced. Reading the 282 codes, it is evident that family and property were very important to those early societies and so was the practice and malpractice of medicine. The practice of medicine has been intertwined with governments and politics ever since the Hammurabi codes in varying degrees.

With the rise of Christianity, the practice of medicine became the domain of the church. The creators of codes of conduct for physicians and the body which admonished physicians and set reimbursement rates were mostly members of the church. With the rise of Islam in the Middle East and its emphasis on scientific discovery and development of scientific bodies, the practice of medicine became more structured and was mostly supervised and influenced by towering scholars such as Razi and Avicenna. During the Reformation and Renaissance, the influence of religious bodies on medicine waned and by the 18th and 19th century, medicine became quite distinct and independent of church doctrine and norms.

With the church's position reduced in Europe's societies, another filled the void to provide guidance and enforcement of rules and norms: The government made its inroads into the practice of medicine. Beginning in the 18th century, some European countries began to collect public health statistics such as infant mortality, longevity, and life expectancy. With increased medical knowledge and the firm understanding of the germ theory of disease, governments became more active in public hygiene campaigns by providing clean water and reducing sewage and manures in the cities. With the help of powerful and capable governments cities became more sanitary and livable and societies improved.

The delivery of health care still, as Hippocrates said some 2,500 years earlier, involved the disease, the patient, and the physician. The relationship between the patient and the physician was very transactional and simple. Patients sought medical advice and treatments based on their desire to seek it and the payments were negotiated between the involved parties. Reputable physicians demanded higher prices and the young and inexperienced physicians demanded much less. There was no single governing body setting rates for treatments and repercussions of malpractice were set by professional guilds, universities, and hospitals which supervised the delivery of care.

It was not until the 19th century that modern governments became involved in medicine and realized the potency and impact on society and one's legacy which has lasted until today. It was in Germany, the leader in medicine and science in the 19th century, where the relationship between government and medicine commenced. The 19th-century Germany produced many memorable people who had an outsized influence on many European nations.

Germany's ascendance started with the elevation of Otto von Bismarck (1815–1898) to prime minister in 1862. He was leading a nation which was not considered a power among European countries and the German-speaking people were dispersed among many countries. Central Europe, where he was the prime minister of Prussia, was not the traditional seat of power and industry. The Austrian Empire and France were more central and important in the power dynamic of Europe. With a sense of purpose and immense skills, after three wars in nine years, von Bismarck was able to unite most of the German-speaking people under one empire and the Second Reich was born. He became the first Imperial Chancellor in 1871 and served in that role until 1890. Once he managed to secure Germany's central role in Europe, he managed to balance European powers to avoid war and maintain German's standing in Europe. He was able to create a framework where Europe was peaceful for twenty years. His skills at diplomacy and war probably eclipsed Klemens von Metternich, the Austrian statesman, who was the quintessential diplomat in the early 19th century.

During the 19th century, Germany was a vibrant place for ideas. Rudolf Virchow, the German physician who pioneered social medicine and public health, was a liberal who opposed many of Bismarck's conservative ideologies and advocated for public health and well-being. He claimed many of society's ills and people's sicknesses could be cured by correct public policy and always pushed for reform. At one point, Virchow's searing criticism of Bismarck prompted the wily Chancellor to challenge Virchow to a duel. It never happened.

Another giant in philosophy and economics in Germany was Karl Marx (1818–1883). His many works, such as *Das Kapital* and *The Communist Manifesto*, painted a picture of German society and much of Europe as a place where the bourgeoise class exploited the working population. Along with his collaborator Friedrich Engels (1820–1895), their arguments about capitalism and the class struggle painted a picture of maltreatment of working people who were losing in the system as designed by their leaders.

Bismarck, who was a conservative policymaker during his rise to power and was against many liberals and revolutionaries, always advocated for the status quo and was not dogmatic in his approach to governing and state power. He was against any actions to disturb the arrangement of Europe when he rose to power. Once he was prime minister, he didn't accept the arrangement where Prussia was weak and became a revolutionary to change the standing of his country to make it a powerful country. Once he achieved his desired outcome, Germany united, powerful, and the center of Europe, he became conservative in his approach and switched from being a warmonger to being a peacemaker to preserve his gains. Bismarck's philosophy was power grab, ascendance, and then preservation of power.

Realizing the revolutionary forces were growing in Europe and the ascendance of Marxism and socialism in his own society, Bismarck set out to counter their influence and prevent them from gaining power in Reichstag. He passed the Anti-Socialist Law in 1878. The law prevented Social Democratic meetings, newspapers, and gatherings.

Having witnessed the short but bloody socialist uprising in France, Bismarck, ever the calculating statesman, was determined to undercut the socialist influence in German society. He considered socialists a threat to what he was able to build by joining many principalities and small regions to form a united Germany. He co-opted the socialist ideas and preempted their agitation in German society. To blunt their arguments against his conservative approach to domestic policy, he proposed some unique and groundbreaking reforms for workers.

In 1883, Bismarck passed *Krankenversicherungsgesetz*, the sickness insurance law to protect workers during sickness. The scheme involved setting up local committees—funded by workers and employers—to cover the cost of medical care for the employees. In 1884, he passed the Accident Insurance law and, in 1889, the Pension and Disability law was introduced into legislation.

These successive laws were meant to thwart the appeal of socialism by allaying workers that were starting to grow increasingly restless during the Industrial Revolution. The health insurance law was mostly for big cities which eventually spread to rural areas as well. The number of participants soared to three million in its first year. The program was very popular with the public.

The sweeping reform was very successful. German emigration prior to the social welfare laws was very high. Young men immigrated to America for work. After the social reforms, emigration to America decreased substantially. People preferred to stay and work in Germany and enjoy the safety net which was unparalleled in any modern society at the time. Bismarck's ability to dent the popularity of socialists was not as successful as the programs he created. By

1912, the Social Democrats were the majority in Reichstag. The programs created a constituency for Social Democrats and, once people realized the benefits of the programs, they wanted to keep politicians who were strong proponents of the programs.

Bismarck was an effective statesman and politician. He was lucky to be chancellor to Wilhelm I who lived to be ninety years old and was very supportive of Bismarck. His long premiership enabled him to experiment and enact laws which could have not been done by a fly-by-night politician. His long, illustrious career gave him the opportunity to enact what was needed to keep German society together in the early stages of the Second Reich.

The Bismarck system prevailed while most of his other achievements were undone by his successors. Wilhelm II, the grandson of Wilhelm I, pursued an ill-advised war with France and England (World War I), undid the state Bismarck had meticulously put together, and the Second Reich ended with the creation of the Weimer Republic in 1919. Bismarck's lasting legacy was his health insurance law which prevailed and became a part of German society's fabric through the Weimar Republic, the rise of the Third Reich (Nazism), and utter annihilation in World War II. The system not only survived in Germany, but it was also exported to France, Belgium, and the Netherlands during the Nazi occupation. The Allies were victorious and were able to kick the Nazis out of their countries, but those countries kept the system which was forced upon them by Nazi occupation. The system flourished in those countries and Bismarck's health insurance reform became his lasting legacy. It did not escape the attention of politicians of many stripes that, to build a legacy, medicine was as important an arena as any foreign policy adventure. In the 20th century, politicians, industrialists, billionaires, capitalists, socialists, religious movements, lawyers, community organizers, and basically any man or woman of ambition dove in head first into the practice and delivery of medicine in hopes of building a legacy.

Bismarck introduced the practice of politics to the art of medicine. Politics became a part of medicine, bringing its gifts and, more importantly, its flaws to the practice of medicine. Flourishing democracies in post-World War II were fertile ground for aspiring parties to attract public support and bring voters to the ballot box by getting involved in the delivery of medicine. Next to religion, medicine is ubiquitous in most societies. The practice of medicine touches almost everyone from birth to death. It became a tempting area for politicians to get engaged and almost political malpractice to ignore it.

The next major involvement of government in medicine occurred in Great Britain. During the destructive World War II when England was constantly bombarded by German planes and the populace was devastated by shortages, killings, and the mayhem that was engulfing the entire continent, the government of Great Britain funded a report for social reform in post-war England. William Beveridge (1879–1963), the British economist and social reformer, was selected to publish the report.

After one year of research, in 1942, Sir Beveridge published his report titled *Social Insurance and Allied Services*. In his report, he identified five "Giant Evils" of British society to combat. The five evils were want, disease, ignorance, squalor, and idleness. This was more like a giant exercise of mental masturbation than identification of realistic problems. It is hard to measure ignorance. Who would be the authority to judge the populace's level of ignorance? Those lofty and utopian ideals and goals were understandably ignored, even if not directly laughed at, during the biggest war England had witnessed. Churchill promptly ignored the whole exercise and the report. However, upon the publication of the report, it was shown to be very popular with the public. A public survey found that 95% of people had heard of the report and many had a positive response to the report.

Politicians, approval-craving creatures, did not ignore it in the post-war period. During the general election of 1945, Labour and Conservative parties agreed on carrying parts of the Beveridge Report, including providing comprehensive medical coverage. England's proposal was a radical idea. The government was going to be the central player in health care, unlike Bismarck's approach of local schemes with government oversight.

The Labour Party won the election of 1945 and the new prime minister, Clement Attlee (1883–1967), introduced the National Health Service legislation and it became the law of the land. On July 5th, 1948, the British health minister, Aneurin Bevan (1897–1960), strode into Park Hospital in Manchester to launch the National Health Service (NHS) and usher in a radical idea in health care. The program brought hospitals, doctors, pharmacists, dentists, opticians, and many other providers under one body, controlled and funded by taxes collected from the masses, and the services free to everyone at the point of service. The hospital which is now called Trafford General Hospital was the birthplace of NHS. *The Manchester Guardian* newspaper had the correct headline, "The Transfer of the Hospitals."

Mr. Bevan walked into the room of an unsuspecting patient, 13-year-old Sylvia Diggory, with photographers in tow to mark the occasion. The picture of the health minister walking in the hospital courtyard with nurses and doctors standing at guard like defeated soldiers saluting the new conqueror was a great illustration of the hubris and folly of the experiment called the NHS. The paper had this caption underneath the photo: "The handing over of this hospital to the Minister was a symbol of the transfer that took place all over the country yesterday."

The newly created board took charge of 2,700 of 3,000 hospitals which were operating in England. It was a great triumph for Beveridge and his vision of a service totally funded by taxpayers, administered by the government, and free to all. The politicians soon realized that health care was not so simple and faced financial problems just a few years after its inception. Changes proposed and enacted to cover some of the skyrocketing expenses led to the resignation of Mr. Bevan in protest.

The NHS has endured and has had triumphs and setbacks. The system which the British adopted did not influence other nations and the model was not adopted the way the Bismarck system was adopted across Europe. I believe the reason the British politicians did not adopt the Bismarck system which was tried for almost a half-century with a good track record was the system's country of origin. It was hard after World War II to adopt a system which Germans created. Just like when Churchill took a sulfa drug, a German creation, and the British newspaper declared incorrectly that Churchill took penicillin, a British discovery. Once politicians became involved in medicine, they brought their taboos, political calculations, talking points, maneuvering, positioning, and quest for maximum recognition and fame.

The basic flaw and shortcoming of the NHS was the way it was created. The lofty and almost juvenile aspiration of the document (to eliminate want, ignorance, and so on) which inspired the creation of the NHS and the publicity-seeking behavior of Bevan at its launch made the whole exercise, not a quest for service to mankind, but a grandiose spectacle to stroke politicians' egos. Bismarck's entreaties into medicine was a calculation to preserve German society and the workers which were needed for many German industries. Bismarck never made any grandiose declaration by launching the program like the creation of the NHS. The Bismarck program started small and evolved and grew organically in German society. Bismarck's success was evident in the number of countries which adopted this German version of health care delivery.

Canada followed a different path than Great Britain. Canada adopted government-funded insurance. In 1984, the Canada Health Act was passed which streamlined the health care system. The government provides health insurance to all, which is funded by taxpayers, and the providers file insurance claims to the regional carriers for payments. The cost of procedures, hospitalizations, and drugs are controlled by the government. The national government sets payment rates for services and medications but the patient and doctor relationship is still not the domain of the government which is a far superior system than the NHS in which every aspect of delivery is the domain of the government.

Since Bismarck, governments in most Western countries have played a role in medicine and the delivery of care. Once statesmen realized the potential impact on their constituents, medicine and politics have been intertwined. One does not exist without the other. They must come to depend on each other to maintain the system whether it is functioning or not. The 20th century was the century where political medicine became the fabric of most societies. In the post-World War II global order (Pax Americana), Western societies experienced a long period of unprecedented peace and prosperity. Their post-war efforts were not geared toward building big armies or conquering neighbors or faraway places. Most politicians' energies and efforts were put into the restructuring of the welfare state.

Western governments designed and maintained elaborate social welfare systems never before seen in human civilization. This contract between governments and their populace produced a new set of rights and expectations which were unheard of a few decades before. The people had a right to health care from the cradle to the grave, as well as pensions and disability payments and so on. The quality and health metrics of Western populations, accordingly, showed marked improvement compared to the rest of the world. In most Western countries, probably the health minister was more important than the foreign minister for the success of any democratically elected government. During the latter half of the 20th century, Western governments tinkered, altered, shaped, revamped, and revolutionized, or any other term you can think of, the delivery of medical care.

American statesmen were not immune to the new temptations of medicine. America eventually immersed itself in the delivery of health care like many Western countries. During the Cold War, every aspect of democracies and communism were compared and contrasted including health care and health outcomes. The communist countries also delved into health care and considered it their main responsibility to equalize their societies' class system. The competition with communism nudged America into the delivery of health care to ensure a better system.

Most state-run medical systems in communist countries were inadequate at best and negligent at worst. The health outcomes were not nearly as impressive as Western democracies. They tampered and fiddled with the health care system to a point that it was not functioning in many communist countries. Some interventions were draconian like Ceausescu, the Romanian dictator who outlawed contraception of any kind in hopes of adding young members to his followers. The opposite happened. The ensuing population surge of young people caused his downfall and his (and his wife's) eventual execution.

The love affair between statesmen and medicine, which was started with Bismarck's actions to blunt the appeal of socialists by creating a health insurance scheme, has lasted for more than a hundred years and shows no sign of abating. The delivery of healthcare has become the cornerstone of many Western democracies and the preoccupation of many Western governments and developing nations. Since Bismarck, medicine and governments have become more entangled and intertwined for good or ill. Medicine ceased to be a compact between the patient and the physician. A new player was thrust into the formula of health care which did not exist a mere century earlier: the government.

Chapter 13

American Health Care

American health care is as unique as the idea of a nation bound by ideology, not common ancestry. Before enlightened men who were versed in human history and civilizations set out to create a nation free of organized religious influence and untethered to any king or queen, countries were created by assembling people of common background and cultures in a continuous land area, usually led by a strongman. America was going to be different than previous civilizations and powers. Franklin and Jefferson were well aware of the previous powers and realized, to make a mark, one had to create an enduring system of government to defy conventional wisdom.

The idea of individual liberty—free of government interference and intrusion—was the basis of declaring independence from Great Britain. The new American system was not going to bow to a person but to an ideology which brought disparate cultures and people together. It was an experiment for certain and no one was sure of its eventual fate. Against high odds, the American Revolution was successful, and a new nation was born which guaranteed individual rights and provided liberty and freedom for people to pursue their dreams with minimal intrusion and micromanagement from the central government.

The same philosophy which created the American experiment in self-governance extended to many fields and areas. Medicine was not immune to the same ideology of freedom to pursue one's own ideas and thoughts. The American medical system started in an organic fashion without any supervision or guidance from the central government in those early days of the republic. Benjamin Rush, the only physician to sign the Declaration of Independence, did not provide or insist on any guidelines or regulations regarding the practice of medicine or education of physicians.

In this free environment, medicine in America evolved in an unregulated and decentralized fashion. A physician's training was mostly done by apprenticeships to local physicians without any requirement for competency. Physicians were not associated with any universities since America lacked any high-caliber medical university. Physicians experimented a lot and were not punished for thinking and practicing differently than the accepted standards of practicing physicians.

It was this unregulated and untraditional environment which produced some positive results. The first women to obtain medical degrees were in the United States. The first abdominal surgery without anesthesia happened in America. The introduction of anesthesia and the first use of the anesthetic gas took place in America. Besides these positive examples of this unregulated environment, many negative consequences were also present. The practice of medicine in America was very substandard and uneven. Since the education of physicians was not uniform across most cities, let alone the whole country, the quality of physicians was also not uniform. There were no licensing bodies to root out bad physicians.

The medical societies or universities were not strong and respected to police practicing physicians. In Europe, the training of physicians was mostly connected to universities with respectable track records. The local physicians' societies strictly regulated the practice of physicians and would deprive any physician of their ability to practice if they did not adhere to local norms and ethics.

Just like the freewheeling nature of medicine in America, the delivery of care was also unregulated and left to localities to figure out. Most people paid the physicians for the care they received, and the price was negotiated by the patients and physicians. The reputable physicians commanded higher payments as opposed to the young and inexperienced physicians. The reputation of the physician among the local population was the key factor in setting the price for care. Just like the disparity in quality of physicians, the price of care was also very uneven in many places.

With the *Flexner Report* in the 1920s, which was discussed earlier, the American medical education was reformed, and the quality of education increased as did the caliber of the physicians. Individual states became involved in regulating the practice of medicine by issuing licenses to qualified physicians thus reducing the number of physicians in each state. The *Flexner Report* also reduced the number of medical schools and graduating physicians further reducing their numbers and increasing the salaries for physicians.

The reforms and transformation of medicine in America were not initiated by the government. The impetus for reforming and regulating the practice of medicine was initiated by wealthy industrialists at the beginning of the 20th century. The American government was still not interested in regulating medicine or get involved in delivering care to its people. American statesmen had other ideas and were preoccupied with other concerns and left medicine to its own devices. Teddy Roosevelt (1858–1919) wanted to expand the Navy, so America could become a superpower. Woodrow Wilson (1856–1924) wanted to create a new world order with his League of Nations and the war to end all wars. Calvin Coolidge (1872–1933) had an allergy to government intervention in most circumstances even in natural disasters.

One group of Americans that the government was concerned with their well-being and was active in ensuring the delivery of medical care was and still is American military veterans. The Continental Congress of 1776 provided pensions and care for soldiers who enlisted in the army to fight the redcoats. This was designed to encourage enlistments to form a standing army to battle Great Britain. After the Revolutionary War, soldiers' homes were established to provide care for the wounded veterans. The Civil War produced many injured and the same commitment to care for the wounded soldiers was evident in the post-Civil War era. The American government became more involved in delivering proper care to wounded soldiers in the wars that ensued. With each war, the injuries were more gruesome, and the care was more specialized. Soon the veterans' homes that cared for soldiers became hospitals run by the United States government to treat wounded soldiers returning from wars abroad. After World War I, which was the first war where tanks and deadly weapons were used including chemical and biological weapons, the United States government enacted laws to create hospitals specifically to care for the returning soldiers because of the specialized care they needed. Congress set aside money to lease private hospitals and for building new hospitals specialized in treating complex war injuries.

World War II—which was more devastating than World War I—the Vietnam War, the First Persian Gulf War, and the Iraq invasion have produced many wounded veterans and the budget to build hospitals and expand services for the veterans grew. The American people have made a moral commitment to care for the soldiers who fight wars and they insist on providing great care for the returning soldiers. This common consensus among Americans has formed the impetus to expand the budget of the Veterans Administration (VA) to build new hospitals and hire more people. The VA hospital system is the second largest bureaucracy after the Pentagon with a budget of almost $200 billion. The VA has become a colossal organization which oversees and runs more than 150 hospitals and 800 clinics.

The VA system is like the British NHS. The hospitals are owned by the government and the physicians and nurses are employed by the government. The VA system is the backbone of medical training in the United States. Many medical students and residents receive part of their training in VA hospitals. The care veterans receive at these hospitals is great if they can get it. As most physicians know, the wait for care is long and the bureaucracy is hard to reform since every aspect of the process is dictated by a central authority with political wrangling and angling, positioning, turf wars, and massive inefficiencies. The employed physicians and caregivers have no incentive to work efficiently and increase their patient volume since everyone is salaried and, if one works harder and treats more patients, he or she takes home the same pay as the one who works the system to treat fewer patients. The wait time at VA hospitals is notoriously long and, even with increased budgets, those long wait times have not gone away. The VA system wastes a lot of money on buying medical equipment. They usually buy the most expensive medical equipment, priced higher than the market, and utilize it less effectively than the private hospitals.

Besides the veteran population, the United States government historically had little role or inclination to get involved in the private health care business. Bismarck changed that calculation by introducing the idea of health insurance in the 1890s and was quickly evident how popular the idea was with the German public when it resulted in reduced emigration and better health metrics in Germany. The United States government was not involved in health care delivery except for delivering health care for veterans. Like many fields in America, the private sector provided a solution for health care delivery. The health insurance scheme started in the 1920s in Dallas, Texas. Baylor University hospitals offered the local teacher association a benefit of twenty-one days of hospital care for a fixed amount which was $6 annually. Blue Cross health insurance was born. The plan proved to be popular and soon other Dallas employers contracted with Baylor to offer the same benefits to their employees. The Blue Cross' health insurance group plans spread all over the country and the idea of paying for care at a fixed price negotiated by a group of individuals became entrenched in the system (and has been a headache for companies' human resource departments ever since).

Blue Cross provided coverage for hospital care. The cost of care at clinics and doctors' offices was not covered by Blue Cross health plans. Another group of employers in the Pacific Northwest contracted with a group of physicians to provide care for their employees. Blue Shield was born. In the 1940s, Blue Shield was providing coverage for physician fees in California and soon throughout the country. Since the government was not involved in the delivery of care in the private sector, the creation of a single health plan to provide comprehensive care was hindered and the delivery and payment of care has fractioned into separate plans. There's been confusion ever since. This is the origin of hospitals and physicians representing different interests and rival associations. The American Medical Association was concerned with physician's payments and the American Hospital Association was interested in protecting their share of the payments. The separation of hospitals and physicians has not led to an efficient "marketplace" where forces reduce costs, but rather an inefficient system with higher costs and unnecessary rivalry. In 1982, Blue Cross and Blue Shield eventually merged, but not before entrenching its ineffective payment system into the broader medical care system (more on this subject later).

The rapid rise of enrollees in private health plans occurred because of a government action which accelerated the rapid rise of private health insurance in the country. During World War II, the United States labor market was very tight. The government enacted wage and price controls to fight off inflation and price gouging. Employers had difficulty attracting workers. Unable to increase the salary of prospective new hires, they turned to fringe benefits to attract new employees. The United States Labor Board agreed with employers that the health care benefits and sick leave were not part of wages (wrong!) and can be offered without violating the wage control clauses. Soon, employers were offering generous health insurance plans to their employees. The public sector also followed the example of private companies and offered health insurance for public sector employees. The private health insurance enrollees exploded in the decades that followed culminating in today's health care environment where approximately 50% of the population receive their health care coverage through employers.

Until 1965, the only part of medical care which concerned the government was the care of veterans. The American government's first major foray into the medical field was in 1965, when Lyndon Johnson introduced Medicare and Medicaid legislation. Franklin Delano Roosevelt tried to include health care coverage as part of a Social Security Act but was not successful. President Truman tried to pass universal health coverage and was not able to muster enough support in Congress. Lyndon Johnson, who was a skilled legislator before becoming president, was able to pass the law to cover many uninsured people. The elderly were not able to buy health coverage in those years because they lacked employment and the cost of insurance was high given their age. They were not able to use the "marketplace" to buy insurance because the marketplace dictated that covering older individuals costed too much money and was not good for business. The poor could not afford the premiums. The government filled a void left by the health insurance industry. The health insurance industry was interested in covering healthy people who did not need as much health care as the older population. The program's first beneficiaries were Mr. and Mrs. Truman. The former president and his wife, Bess, were decent people and never wanted to profit from the office of the presidency during their post-presidential years. They were poor financially but rich in character and didn't even own a home let alone medical insurance. The Trumans were the perfect, first beneficiaries and it was meant to give people in their later years peace of mind that their health needs would be taken care of.

The flaw with Medicare and Medicaid was not its intention but its implementation. Since the government had limited knowledge and skills to administer a health plan, it sought out Blue Cross and Blue Shield to devise the plan. Blue Cross and Blue Shield, not surprisingly, designed a system just like their model—a plan for hospital care, Plan A, and a plan for physicians' services, Plan B—further entrenching their flawed system (Blue Cross and Blue Shield's system) into the broader health care system. The separate plans for separate health care services has resulted in increasing jockeying and turf wars between competing interests, which should be aligned, and, more importantly, it has created inefficient and expensive care.

After President Johnson, many presidents tried to achieve universal coverage and, up to this book's publication, it has not been achieved despite many efforts. Even though Medicare was passed in face of strong opposition from the Republicans, in a short time, it became the third rail of politics and no one dared to challenge it or change it. Medicare and Medicaid became the standard political campaign themes since its passage. Politicians have routinely accused each other of actions to gut the system regardless of the merit of new ideas in the delivery of care. The government added certain other programs to cover more people who could not find coverage in the health care insurance market like the poor, children, and pregnant women.

A fourth system, which has its roots in antiquity, still survived in America. The self-pay model where the sick seek care on his or her own and pays the hospital and physicians from his or her own funds. The problem with this approach is the fractured nature of care, billing, and prices of services which is inflated then drastically discounted for Medicare and private health insurance but not for the individual, self-paying patient. This model is used mostly by people who are unable to find affordable insurance coverage or do not qualify for government insurance plans. This model is unworkable in the current American health care system which has many players performing tasks which should be streamlined but are not and billed for different parts of the same continuous health care event.

For example, a patient presents with an orbital mass, a possible tumor behind the eye. The surgical removal of the tumor is performed and let's say it was a benign lesion. Here is a partial list of entities and fees for this single health care event:

The surgeon's in office consultation fee, CT scan facility fee, radiologist professional fee (for reading the CT), surgeon fee for performing the surgery, physician assistants' fee (if the surgeon needed extra hands), the hospital facility's fee, anesthesiologist's fee, and the pathologist's fee for reading the specimen.

If a patient is uninsured, it is impossible to negotiate with all of these different entities for fair payment. This is not an isolated event in my practice and I have seen many instances over the years. That list was for a patient with a benign lesion. A lymphomatous lesion, which is the most common scenario, has costs for the oncologist, chemotherapy, radiation, and so forth. The Blue Cross and Blue Shield initial model, which was pioneering and eventually adopted by

Medicare and Medicaid, has permeated the whole system, making it one of the least efficient, bloated, expensive, and, most importantly, patient unfriendly and unhelpful health care delivery system in the world.

As of this writing, the private health insurance provided by employers covers more than 150 million people, Medicaid and related programs provide insurance for 65 million individuals, Medicare covers 55 million people followed by 30 million people who are uninsured (the self-pay model), non-employers' private health insurance covers 20 million people, and about 9 million veterans receive care at VA hospitals (the figures are approximate numbers).

In the 21st century, American health care consists of four main systems with contradictory philosophies and agendas to serve (or more accurately ill-serve) the American public. The Veteran Administration hospitals are managed like the NHS of Great Britain. Medicare, Medicaid, and other government plans are like Canada's system, government health insurance plans which have negotiated the payment rates with the hospitals and physicians and funded by taxpayers. The private insurance model is loosely similar to Bismarck's model funded by employers and employees and individuals administered locally. The fourth model is what I call the Byzantine model, individuals pay directly to providers for the cost of the care they receive when they seek it. This collection of four systems gives us the American health care system. It is a system some argue which gives us different approaches to the delivery of care. This argument would be valid if the competing systems produced cost-effective care but the current system certainly does not provide this.

American health care is as unique as the system of governance that created it. It is an amalgamation of competing, disjointed, disparate, and incompatible systems geared to satisfy different approaches to medical care. The health care providers, physicians, and hospitals have created a complex delivery system to satisfy the competing and contradictory system of payments from private insurance companies, government plans, and individuals. The complexity of paying for health care has made the system work for a lot of people who are not involved in the immediate delivery of care but has made the system unbearable for the nurses, physicians, and health care providers.

This collection of health care systems has produced a wide-ranging price for the same care by the same physicians at the same facilities. The payments for the same service depend on the negotiating skills of the administrator or the lobbying group in Washington, D.C. With each "reform" passed by Congress, a new layer of complexity has been added to the system. Since the government became a big player in health care, different interest groups were able to intrude their way into the space by effectively lobbying the state legislative bodies and the U.S. Congress. Each group of professionals who became part of health care introduced their ethos and practices to the art of medicine. The lawyers introduced robust paperwork to protect against most conceivable liabilities, the businessmen introduced ideas to maximize profits, accountants introduced corporate structures to minimize tax burdens, economists introduced monetary incentives to lower costs, so on and so forth. Many of the new players in health care did not conform to the ethos and ethics of medicine because, understandably, they were not familiar with it. The physicians accommodated and altered their norms to accommodate all these new professions and their corresponding cultures into the field of medicine. The same mechanism which produced a competing and confusing health care delivery system created a health care environment with aims and goals which were not in sync and, in many instances, contradictory. The physicians and nurses were not resistant to the changes from all these different professional classes and were too accommodating and acquiescent. In this whole process, medicine ceased to be a compact between the physician and the patient and became a part of the national economic system with too many constituents, political activists, aspiring statesmen, competing ethos, different professional cultures, government agencies, and ever-changing policies. The physicians failed to assimilate these new players and their expertise into a cohesive body with Hippocratic ethics at its core. Too many professions and interests must be appeased which has crowded and distorted the main mission of medicine: to care for the sick and nurture them back to health.

Because of the new players in medicine, the mission of the health care profession has some contradictory aims. The best health care is the one you should never need. Physicians should promote ideas that keep people healthy in the first place so there's no need to seek medical care but that would work against the financial interests of the medical industry. The shameful part of health care is the blatant commercialization with the aim of increasing revenue by promoting overconsumption of health care. Advertising for medical services and drugs accounts for $10 billion annually in a $200 billion advertising industry. Marketing consultants are an important part of pharmaceutical companies, hospitals, and physician's practices. The national companies adhere to some standards in advertising as to not inflate the promises of drugs or medical procedures but they are still predatory in nature. Some local hospitals and physicians engage in blatant false advertising without many repercussions since the government cannot police every ad in every community.

Since the ethical standards of the profession have been married to the ethos of other industries, marketing included, these blatant, self-serving actions by health care providers and pharmaceutical companies have created harm to the public at large by creating demands for medications or procedures which otherwise would have been rarely used. Everyone who watches the nightly news or listens to the radio can attest to the constant advertising for pharmaceutical drugs and medical procedures which has saturated the airwaves and made the news and entertainment industries dependent on those dollars. The media companies, hospitals, physicians who advertise, and pharmaceutical companies all benefit from their advertising schemes by increasing the utilization of medical procedures and medications to the detriment of the patients and the population at large.

The medical industry spends money and energy in another area which affects the practice and delivery of medicine with no benefit to the patient: lobbying the lawmakers to protect their interests. Since the government is the biggest spender in health care in America, it is natural that the medical industry would spend money to massage proposed laws in their favor or kill legislation which harms their bottom line regardless of patient benefits, all packaged in a slogan of patient's safety. In 2017, according to OpenSecrets.org which tracts lobbying expenditure, health care industries accounted for a significant chunk of lobbying dollars in Washington, D.C.

Here is the list of the biggest spenders in 2017:

1. U.S. Chamber of Commerce
2. National of Association of Realtors
3. Business Roundtable
4. Pharmaceutical Research and Manufacturers of America
5. Blue Cross and Blue Shield
6. American Hospital Association
7. American Medical Association

There are many examples of these forces which have entered the medical industry and altered the delivery of care, further complicating a basic human-to-human transaction. Underneath all of these layers of bureaucracies, legislations, and consultants, the basic function of medicine is buried: the patient receiving care based on the sound judgment of the attending physician with the patient's best interest at the center of consideration. Unfortunately, this basic promise from physician to patient and the compact between the two is malfunctioning and not providing the best care for the patient.

Medicine till the late 19th century was still as Hippocrates had envisioned it. Hippocrates famously said the art of medicine consists of the disease, the patient, and the physician, and that was still true in the late 19th century. Medical delivery was confined to churches, charity hospitals, universities, profit-seeking institutions, and independent physicians. The act of medical practice was still small and local without many layers in those days. With the introduction of public policy into the practice of medicine, many segments of society also became involved in the practice of medicine by convincing the policymakers that there was value that they could bring to the practice of medicine to improve the delivery of care. During the 20th century, statesmen, lawyers, economists, accountants, administrators, managers, policy experts, billers, businessmen, marketing experts, financial consultants, strategic advisors, utilization specialists, high-salaried CEOs, private equity owners, investors, and, the latest, information technologists were added to the patient, the physician, and the disease equation.

By the turn of the 21st century, the advances of scientific medicine were a miracle for many and the delivery of care a nightmare for far too many.

CHAPTER 14

THE 21ST CENTURY AND THE ERA OF COPY PASTE MEDICINE, MARKETING, AND FINANCIAL ENGINEERING

At the turn of the 21st century, medicine and its promise were evident in remarkable health outcomes and measures. Over the preceding 100 years, medicine's progress was remarkable and truly miraculous. At the turn of the 20th century, most communicable diseases were fatal, infant mortality was high, common infections claimed many young lives, and life expectancy and longevity was in the forties and fifties respectively. One hundred years later, life expectancy was almost eighty in advanced Western societies and many Asian countries.

During the 20th century, communicable diseases were defeated by mass immunizations and public sanitary measures such as providing clean water and sewer systems. Infections were controlled by the discovery of antibiotics. Chronic diseases, such as hypertension and diabetes, were controlled with medications and altered lifestyles with greater understanding of the pathophysiology of the disease. Cancer, which was a death sentence decades earlier, was successfully treated by radiation, surgery, and chemotherapy.

Surgery's progress was nothing short of miraculous. The trend toward minimal, invasive surgery with quick recovery and outpatient surgeries which required no hospital stay accelerated the safety profile of many surgical procedures. The outcomes and mortality rates drastically improved with sterile techniques and new instrumentations in surgery. X-rays, and later CT scans and MRIs, improved imaging of the interior organs and led to a better understanding of pathology before surgery, which resulted in more targeted and purposeful procedures.

The HIV virus, which had the potential to develop into a major pandemic disease, was successfully controlled and managed. Since the great influenza pandemic of 1918, medical communities have been able to prevent major outbreaks in the face of increasing international and long-distance travel. Most of the world is now connected and, remarkably, a major pandemic has not happened. The vigilance of many international health bodies such as the World Health Organization has been instrumental in coordinating responses and sharing information about local outbreaks.

In the 21st century, many believed that we had entered a new era. The Industrial Age was ending, and the Information Age was beginning. The euphoria regarding technology with its unlimited promise to change the way humans live and interact was consuming everyone's mind and wallet. The emerging technology reshaped many industries (shopping), destroyed some (travel agencies, video rental stores), and altered many more.

Medicine was not immune to the sweeping changes caused by this new technology. Before the year 2000, the tech industry was busy fixing all those computers which were supposed to malfunction at midnight on January 1st, 2000. Everything had to be "Y2K ready" and industries spent massive amounts of money on a fix. January 1st, 2000 arrived without a hint of any cataclysmic event and was like any other day in human civilization.

Post-Y2K, the technology firms turned their attention to industries which had resisted their help. Medicine was one of those industries which had been resistant to the change and was a lucrative and untapped market for the tech industry. The tech industry started their foray into medicine. Initially, the management side of medicine was introduced to the promise of new technology. With powerful computers, billing, scheduling, and collections were automated, and the benefits were evident immediately by reducing the paperwork. The business side of medicine was chump change for the tech industry compared to the 800-pound gorilla in the room: the patient recordkeeping business. The laboratories and radiology departments adopted the technology and the result was a pleasant surprise. Physicians were able to access patients' radiology reports and blood work efficiently. However, physicians and patient interactions were still documented by pen and paper or dictated.

Physicians, who are mostly conservative in nature (experience in medicine makes most physicians conservative), were reluctant to change from a system which had been around for thousands of years to a new, unknown system. The medical community on its own did not adopt the new technology and fall for the promises made by the tech industry. Since medicine (as explained before) was no longer a basic physician and patient interaction but now involved many players, the tech industry switched from convincing physicians about their products to convincing lawmakers about their wonderful inventions to help mankind (for a hefty profit of course).

During the depth of the Great Recession, the tech industry was able to convince the Obama administration, who was enamored by tech, to bribe physicians and hospitals to adopt electronic medical records on a mass scale. Congress passed a stimulus package in 2009 to help the economy which included $44,000 for each physician to adopt electronic medical records. Physicians and hospitals rushed to buy electronic health records to claim their free money from the government.

Most of the early versions of electronic health records were created by tech experts and not medical professionals. The emphasis of the electronic records was not its ability to record the interaction easily but to maximize billing per patient interactions and meet the government's many mandates. The result was a system which made it easy to create long and comprehensive exams with features such as on-click exam, auto populate, copy forward, my normal, and copy paste. The system designed by the tech industry remembered physician's inputs and automatically filled in some areas for the doctor. If you need to know one thing about medicine, nothing is automatic. Every action, surgery, or medication can elicit an unusual response.

Some physicians and nurses were ready for the new system because they grew up with computers, but most were not comfortable or ready. I remember during a training for the electronic records, the physician next to me, who was getting a one-on-one tutorial by the IT department staff, asked what "right click" was. It was going to be a long day for that poor IT guy.

Whether the nurses or physicians were ready, the electronic health record system was rolled out all over the country and adopted in a few, short years. The result was not good for the patients because of the demand for physicians' time which left less time for patient interaction and the difficulty of extracting useful information about a patient in a deluge of repeated and unnecessary information. The electronic records fundamentally changed the way nurses and physicians interacted with patients and divided the attention of health caregivers between patients and the screen.

The government and insurance companies required a multitude of data points for each patient and physician interaction and required its entry before letting the physicians finalize the exam. These programming requirements were designed to make the government, insurance companies, and billing departments happy. To maximize billing and income, the creator of electronic records designed programs with billing and payment in mind to justify their expensive costs and implementation. Therefore, it's easy to make an eight-page-exam (literally) for a mere five-minute physician-patient interaction and, in some instances, with no patient-physician interaction. Physicians were able to log in from anywhere, office, doctor's lounge, home, in pajamas, or in bed and create an exam without setting foot in the hospital.

The electronic records produced many data points for research and administration to assess the productivity of physicians and staff. If a nurse spends most of her time at the bedside taking care of a sick patient and does not enter as many data points, then she is considered less useful because she had idle time per computer program compared with a nurse who has a stable patient with not much need for close monitoring and has time to enter many data points. Productivity and competency are measured by what is entered into the computer, not the actual act of caring for the patient.

Proponents of electronic medical records argue that, with time, the health care providers will be more efficient in entering data and would not take time away from patient interaction. The benefit of quick access to the medical records would eventually outweigh the downsides. However, access to the records is not as easy either. When reviewing charts for a patient in the hospital, the notes of other colleagues and nurses are so long, comprehensive, and very repetitive (a significant amount of copy-pasted material) defeats the whole purpose of quick access. It is very time-consuming to click on each exam by many physicians and nurses who have seen the patient and come up with a clear view of the patient's problems. Among physicians, it is an open secret and a joke about the exams created by these computer programs and the confusion it has created. These programs will get better, but the medical community must stand up to resist any change or scheme to the practice of medicine which results in adverse effects on patients.

The other phenomenon of 21st-century medicine which has consumed and altered the nature of medicine is the blatant commercialization and marketing strategies to maximize profits. It was not long ago when the consensus and accepted code of conduct was to refrain from self-promotion and commercialization of medical service. It was unfathomable and taboo to advertise for a medical service to increase volume. Medicine is at its best when it is needed the least. A successful medical community is preferably a system where not many people require its services. The more people that need medical attention, the more medicine is failing at its core mission. With the advent of immunization, the need to care for all those patients with those diseases disappeared which is a huge success story. But in commercial endeavors and marketing, the more consumers and demand for your product, the more successful the campaign is. These two opposing ethos met in the field of medicine in America and the medical community totally capitulated to the ethos of marketing. Advertising for medical procedures and health care services has soared which accounts for $10 billion in the $200 billion advertising industry. The pharmaceutical companies spend some $3 billion on direct consumer advertising and more than $20 billion for marketing geared toward health care professionals.

The insane amount of money, hospitals, physicians, and pharmaceutical companies pay for marketing is meant to increase consumption of medical services and drugs which is totally contrary to the mission of medicine. Instead of devising a system where people need less medical attention and medications, the health care industry is creating demand for their many products with some questionable benefits. In most advanced and first world countries, advertising for medical services and medications is not allowed because of the harm it can cause. Marketing and advertising in medicine are uniquely American, which has caused mass consumption of medications, ever increasing use of tests and procedures with some devastating results.

The current opioid epidemic in America is the direct result of the commercialization of health care products. The pharmaceutical companies devised schemes to increase usages of narcotics to alleviate pain combined with government regulation which mandated physicians to manage pain effectively has created an iatrogenic and totally preventable epidemic which is ravaging many communities. The opioid epidemic is the medical industry's creation and the medical community is the sole responsible party for this tragedy.

The marketing campaign adopted by the health care industry created demand for health care products and services unlike any other country. The next logical step was to profit from the unending demand and maximize profit. Hospitals, pharmaceutical companies, and physicians descended on Washington, D.C., to limit the changes needed to correct the excesses of their actions. The laws passed by Congress mostly benefited the entrenched and old industries in medicine. The newly passed legislations did not allow for reform but instead moved the chairs around. Any innovation was met with government intervention usually in favor of the industries which benefit greatly from the status quo. With this arrangement protected by the government, the health care industry turned to the next item, increasing the bottom line.

Hospitals turned to financing to create big buildings with huge corner offices for their CEOs to create more traffic for their products whether they were needed or prudent. The non-profit hospitals were also in this business and took advantage of this environment where expansion and increased health care consumption proved financially beneficial. The hospitals bought rivals and other health care facilities and providers to consolidate their positions in their communities. Each acquisition and expansion was introduced to the public as a way of reducing cost and increasing efficiency. The reason for consolidation was not reducing cost but rather increasing the price by increasing their negotiating power.

Health care facilities were taken over by hospitals and, overnight, increased their prices four to five times for offering the same service.

The practice has shown itself to be so lucrative and has attracted private equity to enter the medical field. The returns on investment are so great that hedge funds buy individual physician practices at inflated prices and consolidated them with multiple other, smaller practices to increase their scale. In turn, they do not reduce the price but increase the price for the same services and make hefty returns on their investment.

The inflated prices for the medical services are paid by insurers and patients. Patients have no negotiating power against the hospitals and big physician groups. The main question is why insurance companies agree to pay the inflated prices. This answer is found in the law passed in 2010 to make health care affordable. The law enshrined that health insurance companies can only keep 15% of their total premiums for administration and profits. While 85% of revenues generated by collecting premiums should be spent on health care, if an insurance company does not spend 85% of the premiums on health care, it had to refund the policyholders.

Therefore, the simple logic for health insurance companies was to increase payments to hospitals and health care providers. Health insurance companies became a commission business. To increase the profits, the insurance companies had to increase spending on health care. The more money they spent on health care, the higher their profits were. The insurance companies agreed to ever-higher demands for payments by hospitals and health care providers and just passed along the higher cost to the patients and their employers while their profits increased because they were collecting more premiums.

The hospitals, health care providers, pharmaceutical companies, and insurance companies all benefited from higher prices for drugs and medical services. The system works for everyone but the patients, employers, and taxpayers.

The American health care system is composed of ill-fitting models which have managed to have many scientific breakthroughs. The innovation in health care procedures and monitoring should make the care less expensive, not more. Medicine in America is a tale of two competing and contradictory realities. The scientific part of medicine is wonderful and the diseases which can be effectively treated are growing by the day. Chronic conditions are treated well, and surgery has progressed to a minimal invasive phase with, in many instances, no hospital stays. Patients are able to be monitored at home or place of work. Telemedicine can bring the health care provider to the patient and answer basic concerns and questions.

The other reality is the motive to maximize profits from all these new innovations which cannot be squared with the mission of medicine. If hospitals, health care providers, and pharmaceutical companies adopt these innovations to reduce people's reliance on physicians, hospitals, and drugs then this scenario will run afoul of the financial and marketing mission of increasing volume and consumption of medicine. Medicine is moving toward outpatient treatment, yet hospitals borrow vast sums of money to build new hospitals with schemes to fill the beds with patients just like a hotel. The new debt needs to be serviced and paid back and the hospitals will create new demand for their products and services by advertising in the community about their latest building and medical equipment whether they are needed or effective. The hospital down the street cannot be left out or risk losing its market share to the competing hospital so it will engage in raising funds to buy the latest gadget and constructing a fancier building, which I can certainly tell you will not improve health outcomes. For the hospitals, acquiring physician practices, buying new equipment, and building gleaming towers has become the new arms race. In the process, the cost of care has become expensive and, more importantly, the outcomes have not improved. In fact, life expectancy in America has suffered a decline for three consecutive years with higher health care spending. The expenditures and priorities have not resulted in a better system with better health outcomes.

Through this metamorphosis of medicine in America, physicians were first reluctant and skeptical and, by the end, were absorbed into this process and became active participants. Physicians as a group did not assimilate the other competing ethics into a cohesive body with patient care at its core. The other factions, financial experts, marketers, and others were more convincing and had more sway to change health care from what has always been a compact between a physician and a patient into an industrial complex. Medicine is run by high-priced CEOs with big corner offices unfamiliar with medicines' history and its unique mission. I have attended meetings where the topics of discussion are led by finance majors. The blatant profit motives are not hidden behind the slogans of service to mankind anymore. It's the rallying cry for many health care institutions.

Physicians accepted other participants' definition of medicine and were willing partners to change it to what is today. The reason why physicians acquiesced to the arrangement was because of the tremendous benefit they received from the new system. American physicians became the most highly compensated profession in America and worldwide. In the process, physicians lost control of the system which has turned against them by labeling physicians greedy and the cause of the high cost of care.

The mission and practice of medicine is clear and simple. At its core is what Hippocrates said millennia earlier: It consists of the disease, the patient, and the physician. To gain the trust of the patient is the highest responsibility of the physician and he or she should act in the best interest of the patient. It is hard to argue that the current system has this ethic at its core. There are too many meetings, discussions, and symposiums in medicine where the patient's interest is not even mentioned.

To accept this system the way it's currently administered is a disservice to the patients. Nurses and physicians—who are the backbone of the health care system—should start challenging and questioning the practices of the system that are not guided by the core mission of medicine: to care, heal, and nurture people back to health so they never need our services.

CHAPTER 15

GLOBAL HEALTH CARE FINANCING

Health care financing is an integral part of medicine in the 21st century. Medicine is financed in a variety of ways. The dominant force in health care financing is, unsurprisingly, the government. Ever since Bismarck started the scheme to finance health care spending, governments, especially Western governments, have become more involved and have assumed a significant burden of the cost. Since there is a wide variation in national income among nations, health care financing is different in many places on Earth. It is crucial to examine the way health care is financed so the system can be recalibrated to fulfill the ultimate mission of medicine. This subject is covered reluctantly because medicine should be about the patients, innovators, and healers but financial consideration is a large part of medicine and it would be a dereliction of duty if the financing part of medicine was not studied and examined.

Countries with low gross national product tend to lack proper financing by central governments. There are two main sources of funds for health care spending. Much of the burden is placed on the patients. Patients spend their own money to pay for health care. The second source of funds are global funds such as the World Health Organization which collects money from Western countries and spends the money in low-income countries. There are some forms of private insurance and government programs, but the contribution from these two sources are minor and not adequate for most of the people.

Patients in these countries seek health care when it's necessary. The emphasis on routine care and prevention is lacking. Patients mostly negotiate directly with health care providers for their services. The health care services in these countries vary greatly from high quality to barely adequate. The upper echelons of society get their basic care in the country and, for more advanced care, they travel abroad for more specialized treatments. The majority of people rely on local health care providers. Non-profit organizations do a good job of providing funds and some provide training which is even more crucial.

The main disadvantage of development assistance provided by international organizations is its delivery method. Some of the funds are transferred to local governments to administer a program. Corruption at local levels is high, and the funds are sometimes diverted to other priorities and fail to reach its intended beneficiaries. The organizations which use the funds to set up hospitals and treatment centers and train the local physicians are more effective and their effects are not evanescent.

The health outcomes and health metrics in low GDP countries are very unsatisfactory. The emphasis is on acute care and infectious diseases. Chronic medical conditions are treated inadequately, and the patients have few rights. The standard of medicine varies greatly in different parts of the country. Regulations to ensure proper training and licensing are minimal. The focus of many international organizations in these countries is childhood immunizations, maternity care, and infectious diseases. The health care needs and problems beyond that are never addressed properly because of the corruption of local authorities. Patients truly suffer in these countries.

When countries advance and become more prosperous, the health care financing changes as well. One big disadvantage when countries move up the economic scale is the reduction of assistance from health organizations. In these developing countries, the burden of health care is shifted back to the patients. Once countries develop economically, international organizations reduce the financial assistance for health care needs. The central governments in these countries are not advanced enough to care for their population and the burden of health care financing is shifted drastically toward the patients. Patients have more money to spend and reluctantly assume the responsibility. Governments increase their spending on health care but not significantly enough to replace the development assistance funds.

Health care standards improve in these countries. Access to technology is enhanced and physicians' training improves. The health outcomes improve as well. Longevity and lifespan increase along with a country's GDP. Central governments assume more of the responsibility to enforce health standards and require licensing and proper training. Health care emphasis shifts from infectious disease and acute care to treatment of chronic conditions like diabetes and hypertension. The transition to developing nation is sometimes not pleasant for the patients. While advanced care is available in the country, access to it is spotty and the cost of care prevents many from seeking advanced care for their condition. Government oversight is not enough to ensure uniform access to certain technologies. Populations in big cities benefit more than rural parts of these countries. The cost of care, which is significantly financed by patients, limits access.

As a nation's income increases, more is spent on health care. Once new technologies and advanced treatments are available, patients utilize it and thus spend more on health care. Once the basic needs of man are met, like shelter, food, and safety, it is natural for people to care more about their health and longevity. Health care spending increases as the national gross domestic product increases.

The most notable development when a middle-income country progresses to a high-income country is the formation of private insurance markets. In middle-income countries, patients and governments account for more than 80% of health care spending. In high-income countries, almost a quarter of health care spending comes from private insurance plans. The development of private insurance plans along with significant reduction in patient spending and increased government spending are the hallmarks of a nation's advancement toward being a developed country.

In high-income countries, governments assume a significant role in health care. The majority of health care spending is done by the government and the patient's share of health care spending drastically decreases. Health care spending is no longer dependent on the patient's pocket or his or her negotiation skills. Price negotiations with health care providers are done by private health plans and the government. Patient protection and rights are numerous, and the quality of care is high with higher health care outcomes.

The majority of the funds in advanced countries are spent on chronic conditions such as diabetes and hypertension. The emphasis on infectious diseases is lessened and acute care is a smaller portion of health care spending. One notable difference between developed nations and developing nations is the spending on long-term care. Populations in advanced societies have a higher life expectancy and longevity which produces its own challenges. In some advanced societies, long-term care consumes 20% of total health care spending. In low-income and developing countries, the burden of this portion of health care is usually assumed by family members and friends.

Health care spending is highest in developed countries. People seek the best treatments and access to advanced technologies makes health care more expensive. A bigger share of a nation's income is spent on health care. Health care spending as a share of GDP doubles in high-income nations. Since most of the health care financing is done by the government and private health insurance companies, the natural tendency to seek cost-effective care by patients is reduced. Most patients do not know the cost of care they receive and demand more care in a belief that more care is better for health (not true).

The countries which spend the most on health care per capita are the United States and Switzerland. The United States spends approximately $9,403 per person on health care. Health care spending consumes 17% of gross national product. Approximately 45% of spending is done by the government, 45% by private health insurance companies, and 10% by patients.

America spends almost twice as much per capita on health care than all other high-income countries. The high rate of health care spending cannot be explained by the demography of the United States. Among the eleven high-income countries, America has the lowest ratio of population over sixty-five years of age—14.5%—compared with Japan and Germany with 25% and 21% respectively. Yet Japan and Germany spend $3,727 and $5,182 per person on health care. America's population has the highest rate of obesity, the lowest rate of smokers, high population diversity, and high poverty rate which makes America different from other high-income countries. This, in turn, accounts for some of the higher costs of care, but it still does not account for the doubling of the cost. There are three areas where America's health care spending deviates from other countries and where reforms would make the system more efficient and cost-effective.

In America, the physician and nurse workforce was lower than average among the high-income countries. The composition of specialists to generalists was similar to the group of high-income countries. The glaring difference was the compensation of the physicians and nurses. Nurses deserve better compensation given their significant contribution to health care. America's specialists and generalists earn almost twice as much as their counterparts in other high-income countries. Given the higher cost of education and longer, rigorous training in America, higher income compared to other countries is warranted but almost doubling the income is a difficult argument to make.

Overutilization is also a factor in increased health care spending in America. Cataract surgery volume per 100,000 people is 1,110 in America. The average cataract surgery volume per 100,000 is 971 for the eleven high-income countries and the average percentage of population over sixty-five is 18%. America's share of population over sixty-five is 14%. Cataract surgery is mostly performed on patients over sixty-five. Looking at the numbers, one might mistakenly conclude that utilization is similar in America than other nations. But since America's population of over sixty-five-year-olds is less than other countries, the rate of cataract surgery should be lower not the same or higher. America has some of the highest rates of Caesarian deliveries, magnetic resonance imaging (MRI), computed tomography (CT scans), and total knee replacements.

Another area of American health care which is different is the expenditure on administrative tasks. It is estimated that almost 8% of the cost of care is attributed to administrative expenses. The average administrative cost of care in the other high-income countries is 3%. The 8% figure does not include the countless hours physicians and nurses spend on administrative work which takes time away from direct patient care. The main reason for physician burn-out in today's medicine is administrative work mandated by new regulations and electronic records. The problem has become so acute that many hospitals are appointing wellness officers to address the physician burn-out phenomena. America's health care system always adds another layer or officer to address the latest unintended consequence instead of dealing with the root cause. I am sure the wellness officer will need an office, large staff, and a bunch of long, fruitless meetings to come up with pointless recommendations to treat the symptom instead of the disease.

The last area which makes the American system different and more expensive is the cost of medications. America spends $1,443 per person on medications compared to the average of $749 spent by other nations. Americans use generic medications more than other countries yet the expenditure on medications is still higher. It is estimated that generic medication utilization accounts for 84% of the volume in America compared to the average of 58% for other high-income countries. Americans use generic medication at a (much) higher rate than other countries yet the country pays more for medications. The reason for the discrepancy is that medications which are not generic have a much higher price in America. Since the cost of brand-name medications is so high in America, physicians and patients are utilizing generic medications more frequently thus reducing the market for brand-name medications. The pharmaceutical companies to make up for the loss of volume keep raising the prices of brand-name medications to make up the difference so their quarterly earnings reports look good.

For example, Advair (asthma medication) costs $155 in America compared to the average price of $64 in other countries. In Australia, Advair costs $29. The physicians prescribe it more frequently and patients have no problem buying it at the price of $29 to treat their symptoms. But at $155, insurance companies, physicians, and families look for less expensive alternatives before buying the expensive Advair reducing the sale volume of the medication. Reduced sales volume is met with increasing prices to make up the shortfall in the bottom line. The reason pharmaceutical companies can do this kind of pricing practice in America when price information is readily available online is simply because they can. There is no meaningful overseeing body which prevents them from engaging in this kind of behavior.

America spends more on health care, yet the health care outcomes are not better than most Western countries. Health care metrics have been stagnating or, in some instances, declining in

America lately. One study showed life expectancy among whites in America declining for the first time. More spending has not translated to better outcomes. There is emerging evidence to suggest that increased health care spending and utilization have detrimental effects on health. The opioid crisis is one glaring example. Overutilization of health care and pharmaceutical products caused and is still causing a societal calamity and a public health crisis. The opioid crisis is the sole responsibility of the health care industry in America.

America has the highest maternal mortality rate, infant mortality rate, and neonatal mortality rate compared to other high-income nations. The maternal mortality rate of 26.4 deaths per 100,000 is 2.5 times higher than the next highest rate among the eleven countries. Americans have the lowest life expectancy at birth and health-adjusted life expectancy among the same eleven countries. Some of these statistics are alarming and more spending is not the solution as advocated by many policymakers. A fundamental rethinking of health care delivery and health in general is warranted.

The four basic sources of health care financing which consists of domestic government spending, patient's own funds, private health insurance, and developmental organizations are the backbone of global health care financing. The key question for policymakers and architects of health care financing is what the right combination of these sources should be to achieve the best health care outcome in a cost-efficient manner. For most societies, governments, patients, and private health insurance funds are the main sources of health care spending. The search for the right combination and delivery mechanism has consumed many minds, research papers, symposiums, and think tank organizations with no satisfying conclusion. The goal is to deliver care to everyone who desires it in an efficient manner that does not bankrupt the patient or the nation. The search for the right balance and the combination of the four sources of health care financing goes a long way toward fulfilling the mission of medicine. The search continues, and health care providers should engage in the endeavor because it ultimately affects patients and their families.

Chapter 16

Seeking Balance Between Hippocrates and Modern Forces

Medicine's roots began with *Homo sapiens* emerging and organizing tribal structure. In those early years of human existence, some form of medicine was practiced. Childbirth and caring for infant offspring definitely required a set of skills to ensure the survival of the infant and the mother during the delivery and the first year of life. Naturally, the early physicians were women who cared for their offspring and assisted each other in delivery of their babies. Once human interaction and association with each other increased, skilled labor was created in many fields, and medicine was no exception.

With the creation of civilizations in Mesopotamia, the expansion of cities, and greater concentration of humans in one place, the profession of physician became an integral part of any early society. It is notable that, in those early civilizations in Mesopotamia and Egypt, women healers were present in significant numbers. The women healers like other healers in those early days of human civilization came in many forms such as magicians, witch doctors, spiritual healers, and so on. The women were an integral part of the profession of healing.

With the emergence of Greek civilization and the sophistication of city life in Greece, the profession of medicine evolved. Hippocrates introduced ethics, professionality, and standards to the practice of medicine. His code of conduct for anyone claiming to be a physician forced the profession to become respected among some members of the society and, with time, earned the respect of the wider population.

The downside of the Hippocratic reform was its exclusion of women from the practice of medicine. With the ascendency of Western civilization and its eventual scientific discoveries during the Renaissance, the tradition of the male physician was entrenched in many parts of the world. Medicine suffered from a lack of perspective and insight provided by female healers for millennia. Women were excluded from being physicians but were still instrumental in some monumental contributions such as Lady Mary and Nightingale. It was not until the 19th century in the New World (and initially lacking the rigid structure of Europe) that the first female physician graduated from medical school.

Despite Hippocrates' major flaw which excluded women from the practice of medicine, ethics and humanity made physicians different than other healers. The medicine practiced by Hippocratic physicians was a compact between the patient and the physician with the interest of the patient at the heart of the relationship. There was no question where the loyalty of the physician should lie when treating a patient. Hippocratic medicine lacked scientific rigor and, compared to today's standard, is somewhat akin to voodoo. But given the medical knowledge during that period of human civilization, Hippocrates was able to provide care for his patients with the goal of not harming them by performing unproven and risky procedures. It was a noble goal which is still true today.

Galen, the giant of medicine for fifteen centuries, greatly enhanced Hippocrates' influence and place in medicine. If it was not for Galen, Hippocrates would not have been the important figure he is today. During the early part of the first millennium, Galen's energy and efforts united the medical community around the practice of Hippocratic medicine as practiced and understood by him (Galen). Galen's method was practiced until the Renaissance when new discoveries and enlightened figures such as Vesalius made Galen's medicine unusable.

During the second half of the second millennium, when Western Christian civilization emerged from the Dark Ages and settled their thirty-year religious war in Westphalia, medicine was radically transformed. Discoveries and scientific breakthroughs reshaped the practice of medicine and medicine became more scientific. Life expectancy and longevity markedly increased during the 20th century. Mankind greatly benefited from the advance of medicine and medicine came to be defined by Western standards. The medicine practiced in Africa and Asia lacked the depth and breadth of understanding of pathophysiology and lacked clear benefit to the patients. The African and Asian healers subsequently lost their influence and place in the medical community and the world adopted Western medicine as the gold standard and accepted approach to healing.

The promise of medicine became a reality during the 20th century when new drugs and technology made the practice of medicine more of a science than an art. X-rays, CT scans, and MRIs opened a window into living humans and made diagnosis easier creating a new array of treatments and surgeries to cure some diseases which had been around since humans emerged. By the turn of the 21st century, medicine was a miracle and the benefits of its three-thousand-year odyssey were evident.

The intrusion of other members of society into medicine which started in the late 19th century accelerated during the early part of this century. Medicine became more and more the domain of governments and big businesses. The benefits of successful health care delivery became evident to political parties. The business community realized the potential profits in medicine and rushed in to make those potential gains a reality. In the process, the ethos of medicine yielded to the ethos of government, business, and many other professions. Medicine became a conflicted and confused enterprise without a clear mission statement.

It is in this environment where a leading investment bank explicitly asks, "Is curing patients a sustainable business model?" The prospect of profiting from people's misery is now a thriving business model which should be considered the low point of today's medicine. Physicians were worried about socialized medicine, but no one thought that capitalized medicine could be as bad.

A leading physician staffing company which is listed in the stock market released their quarterly report—a great document save for its glaring omission of the word patient until late in the press release. It is well-worth reading:

"Our results for the first quarter of 2018 build on the momentum we established at the end of 2017, with our focus on operational improvements beginning to bear fruit towards our goal of realizing $50 million in operational efficiencies in 2018 and anticipated run-rate savings of $100 million," said Christopher A. Holden, President and Chief Executive Officer of Envision. "We made significant strides to align our practice support and corporate overhead to support our clinical programs and these efforts contributed to our solid financial results in the quarter. We expect the impact of these efforts to accelerate through the remainder of 2018. We are also making good progress in improving our revenue cycle functions to achieve operational efficiencies, which we expect to realize during the second half of this year. We are also advancing several initiatives to improve the efficiency of our clinical teams as they care for **patients**.

"Our operational focus will be key to our ability to optimize shareholder value as our clinical providers and operations professionals are continuously working to improve **patient** safety, quality and efficiency to deliver value to health systems and the **patients** we serve. We continue to successfully execute on a clearly defined strategy that supports our clinical providers as they participate in high-performing healthcare networks in communities across the country. Our Physician Services' growth validates this strategy."

It is basic nonsense (medical nonsense) that consumes many meeting minutes and talent that would be better used in direct patient care. Investors have a right to make a return on their investment, but the field of medicine is unlike other fields. The mission of medicine is to design systems and behavior where the services of the medical community are not needed. The best medicine is the one which is not needed. Unfortunately, people get sick and need medical services and hopefully the care needed is provided expeditiously so the individual can return to a normal life and not become trapped in the medical system with repeated tests and visits. Far too many times, a patient's interaction with the medical system becomes an ongoing saga with no conclusion. The mission of medicine should consist of making people less reliant on medical services and medications, not ongoing "monitoring,", perpetual appointments, and a steady dose of multiplying medications.

Therefore, the investors and business partners in medicine should realize that the investment will not always produce the desired return or maybe become a lost investment. The core mission of medicine is an antithesis to the interest of these investors. The mission of medicine is not to make handsome returns for investors but, unfortunately, this author has been to too many meetings where financial consideration was front and center of the gathering, not patients' interest.

The new frontier of medical cures which involve gene therapy has shown great promise such as Gilead Sciences' Hepatitis C medications and promises to be as important as the discovery of penicillin and immunization. However, the economics of medicine has distorted the practice of medicine. New discoveries which cure diseases are judged to be bad investments.

Gilead Sciences' Hepatitis C treatment costs around $100,000. With cure rates of 90% for Hepatitis C, the medication was a smashing success. The total revenue of the medication was $12 billion in 2015. The 2018 sales will be around $4 billion. The medical success of the new medication was hailed by the medical community as an example of new science and technology to cure, not merely manage, the disease, fulfilling medicine's promise. Yet the medical success of the breakthrough was greeted with headlines similar to this on MarketWatch.com: "Gilead cured hepatitis C. That's become its biggest problem."

The problem with curing disease was met with this analysis from a Goldman Sachs analyst:

> GILD is a case in point, where the success of its hepatitis C franchise has gradually exhausted the available pool of treatable patients…In the case of infectious diseases such as hepatitis C, curing existing patients also decreases the number of carriers able to transmit the virus to new patients, thus the incident pool also declines … Where an incident pool remains stable (e.g., in cancer) the potential for a cure poses less risk to the sustainability of a franchise.

When Koch and Pasteur were toiling in their laboratories to cure diseases far more widespread and devastating, these considerations such as "franchise" and steady consumers for their products were not the focus or even mentioned. Medicine has come far and low to engage in this kind of dialogue about people's miseries and afflictions.

This economic reality in the pharmaceutical industry has led to many new medications introduced to a marketplace which are not new but rather a modification of what is already available. There are too many copycat medications produced by the pharmaceutical industry to take market shares away from a rival company's existing medication. As the financial analyst clearly mentioned, it is better to have "franchises" which has a large steady pool of patients to take the medication forever. As long as pharmaceutical companies are rewarded for their copycat medications, they will produce these medications which are not breakthroughs and, frankly, in many instances not needed.

The technology revolution which has reshaped many industries has finally entered the medical profession. It has many promises but currently we are in a trial-and-error phase with mixed results. The rapid adoption of electronic medical records is a case in point which has led to overbilling and producing repetitive, useless information. With time, trial, and the new generation which is more comfortable with the technology, the use of technology will improve among health care professionals.

The tech industry, high on their accomplishments and revolutionary reshaping of many industries, has turned to health care as the next front for their battle to reshape existing industries. Their vaulted artificial intelligence, algorithm, and robotics promise to be revolutionary in medicine, or so they say. Just like the Gilded Age where many wealthy robber-barons reshaped medicine a hundred years ago, the current crop of ultra-wealthy tech entrepreneurs is wading into medicine with grandiose desires to reshape it. Unlike Carnegie and Rockefeller, the new robber-barons want to be in the driver's seat steering the industry where they think it should go. They might be correct and what they design might be superior to today's medicine. However, the successful reforms initiated by Carnegie's endowment and Rockefeller's generosity were steered by people with medical and educational backgrounds. Carnegie and Rockefeller provided the funds and the Flexner brothers led the fight to reform and reimagine health care in America which has endured for more than a century. Carnegie and Rockefeller trusted the professionals in the field of education and medicine to lead the effort to design a system. The current robber-barons would be wise to follow the example of other monopolists and realize their limitations in certain fields such as medicine.

Many experts, physicians, patients, and others agree that the medical system needs reform, and some would argue radical reform. The system which was designed a hundred years ago in America by the Flexner brothers has run its course. During the ensuing years, many layers were added to the original framework and the cracks in the system are showing. The American health care system is expensive and, most importantly, does not serve many patients well. Patients' distrust and skepticisms of the medical system is widespread among many sects of society.

The quality of nurses and physicians serving the people has dramatically increased over the past decades. The training is very rigorous, and the graduating physicians are well-prepared to enter the medical field and provide high-quality care. But, unfortunately, the system distorts their training by incentivizing them into practicing volume-based medicine. The way physicians get compensated based on procedures and exams has really done damage to the profession and resulted in a loss of trust from the public. Medicare, which institutionalized this fee-for-service approach has been at the forefront of distorting patient care with its unlimited payments for any exam or procedure. Hospitals, ambulatory surgery centers, physicians' offices, and nursing homes have all joined in to extract as much out of Medicare as possible. With more than a million entities which can bill Medicare, it is no wonder Medicare is the epicenter of many medical fraud cases. It is time to look at every level of care and finance to reform the current system. There is enough money in the system to care for everyone in the United States and have money left over for other priorities.

One of the great discoveries of the 20th century which has not fully realized its promise is the discovery of DNA's structure. The process of the discovery was many decades in the making, but the bulk of the recognition went to two young scientists, one American and one British. DNA was first described in 1869 by a Swiss chemist, Friedrich Miescher (1844–1895). His work on white blood cells led to the discovery of nucleic acids which would eventually be named deoxyribonucleic acid (DNA).

Many decades later in the 20th century, the interest in Miescher's research was rekindled. Russian biochemist Phoebus Levene's (1869–1940) research further illuminated the structure of DNA. A great breakthrough occurred when Austrian researcher Erwin Chargaf (1905–2002), inspired by published research on genes by the Rockefeller Institute, discovered the basic composition of DNA material. In 1953, James Watson (1928–, age 90) and Francis Crick (1916–2004) aided by research done by two English researchers, Rosalind Franklin (1920–1958) and Maurice Wilkins (1916–2004), and Chargaf's findings put the pieces of the puzzle together. Watson and Crick discovered the double-stranded helix structure of DNA and opened the door for an endless and promising area of medicine. The future of medicine which many believe lies in the promising discoveries in gene therapy will transform the practice of medicine and subsequently benefit countless patients.

The future of medicine is bright and exciting. It is a great time to be in the field of medicine. In ten to twenty years, many assumptions and practices by the medical community might become obsolete and will go the way of bloodletting. The promise of robotics and artificial intelligence is still in its infancy. These new frontiers can come together to create a great health care experience for the patients and benefit mankind in general. However, all the exciting discoveries which lie ahead are not sufficient if prudency, ethics, and the art of medicine are lost along the way.

New artificial intelligence programs can diagnose many diseases and provide treatments somewhat accurately, but it cannot allay the fear of the patient or provide calming guidance and compassion for the afflicted. As many physicians can attest, Google has scared many people into physicians' offices for perspective and reassurance. Whatever the future brings, it will be exciting and revolutionary, but the basic principles of Hippocratic medicine cannot be lost in the euphoria of new technologies and treatments. Medicine will progress forward, but there is no progress from the basic ethos of medicine which is to comfort the afflicted, nurture the sick back to health, and advocate for treatment options with the best interest of the patient at the center of the equation with other considerations as non-factors.

After thousands of years, medicine is still as basic as it started. Medicine is a compact between the patient and the physician with the interests of the patient at its center. The only change in medicine from those early years is the armament of treatments which can be offered to patients. Medicine would be wise to never lose sight of its original mission, which is to gain the trust of the patient, heal, and care for the infirmed without the influence of other forces that have multiplied over the decades. If medicine abides by its guiding principles beautifully enunciated 3,000 years ago, the future will have endless promising possibilities for the true focus of medicine: patients. The practice of medicine is a promise made many moons ago by Hippocrates and his many followers through the millennia to the infirmed to provide care and healing with the safest, cutting-edge treatments guided by Hippocratic ethics. Medicine has always been and will always be an art, mastered by the ones who believe in its core mission.

Select Bibliography

Affairs., Department of Veterans. "About VA." *History of VA*, 1 Jan. 2005, www.va.gov/about_va/vahistory.asp.

Boissoneault, Lorraine. "Bismarck Tried to End Socialism's Grip-By Offering Government Healthcare." *Smithsonian.com*, Smithsonian Institution, 14 July 2017, www.smithsonianmag.com/history/bismarck-tried-end-socialisms-grip-offering-government-healthcare-180964064/.

Boyd, Robert, and Joan B. Silk. *How Humans Evolved*. W. W. Norton & Company, 2018.

Braudel, Fernand, and Richard Mayne. *A History of Civilizations*. Penguin Books, 2005.

Campbell, Denis. "Nye Bevan's Dream: a History of the NHS." *The Guardian*, 18 Jan. 2016.

Celsus, Aulus Cornelius. *On Medicine*. Harvard Univ. Press, 2007.

Collaborators, Network. "Evolution and Patterns of Global Health Financing 1995–2014: Developmental Assistance for Health, and Government, Prepaid Private, and out-of-Pocket Health Spending in 184 Countries." *The Lancet*, vol. 389, no. 10083, 2017, pp. 1981–2004.

Cunningham, Andrew, and Perry Williams. *The Laboratory Revolution in Medicine*. Cambridge University Press, 1992.

Debus, Allen G. *Chemistry, Alchemy and the New Philosophy, 1550–1700: Studies in the History of Science and Medicine.* Variorum Reprints, 1987.

Debus, Allen G. *Paracelsus, Five Hundred Years: Three American Exhibits.* Published by the Friends of the National Library of Medicine, Inc. for the Hahnemann University Library, the National Library of Medicine, and the Washington University School of Medicine (St. Louis), 1993.

Debus, Allen George. *Chemistry and Medical Debate: Van Helmont to Boerhaave.* Science History, 2001.

Diamond, Jared M. *Guns, Germs, and Steel: the Fates of Human Societies.* Norton, 2011.

Elgood, Cyril. *A Medical History of Persia: and the Eastern Caliphate, from the Earliest Times until the Year A.D. 1932.* At the Univ. Press, 1951.

Flexner, Abraham. *Medical Education in the United States and Canada: A Report to the Carnegie Foundation for the Advancement of Teaching.* Carnegie Foundation, 1910, pp. 1–346, *Medical Education in the United States and Canada: A Report to the Carnegie Foundation for the Advancement of Teaching.*

Geison, Gerald L. *Private Science of Louis Pasteur.* Princeton University Pres, 2016.

Gill, Gillian. *Nightingales: the Extraordinary Upbringing and Curious Life of Miss Florence Nightingale.* Random House Trade Paperbacks, 2005.

"Gilman's Inaugural Address." *Johns Hopkins University,* www.jhu.edu/about/history/gilman-address/.

Goldberg, Herbert S. *Hippocrates, Father of Medicine.* Authors Choice Press, 2006.

Gradmann, Christoph, and Elborg Forster. *Laboratory Disease: Robert Koch's Medical Bacteriology.* Johns Hopkins University Press, 2009.

Grundy, Isobel. *Lady Mary Wortley Montagu.* Oxford Univ. Press, 2004.

Gruner, Cameron. *The Canon of Medicine of Avicenna; Adapted by Laleh Bakhtiar from Translation of Volume 1 by O. Cameron Gruner and Mazhar H. Shah:* Kazi Publications, 2014.

Harari, Yuval N., et al. *Sapiens: a Brief History of Humankind.* Harper Perennial, 2018.

Hippocrates, et al. *Hippocratic Writings.* Penguin, 1987.

Johns Hopkins Magazine, pages.jh.edu/~gazette/1999/jan0499/obit.html.

Jones, Alexander Raymond. "Ptolemy." *Encyclopedia Britannica,* Encyclopedia Britannica, Inc., 11 May 2017, www.britannica.com/biography/Ptolemy.

King, L.W. *The Code of Hammurabi,* Yale Law School, 2018, avalon.law.yale.edu/ancient/hamframe.asp.

Kristof, Nicholas. "Unmasking Horror." *The New York Times,* 17 Mar. 1995.

Kyle, R. A. "Gerhard Domagk." *JAMA: The Journal of the American Medical Association,* vol. 247, no. 18, 1982, pp. 2581–2581., doi:10.1001/jama.247.18.2581.

Lindemann, Mary. *Medicine and Society in Early Modern Europe.* Cambridge University Press, 2010.

Lister, J. "An Address on the Antiseptic System of Treatment in Surgery." *Bmj,* vol. 2, no. 394, 1868, pp. 53–56., doi:10.1136/bmj.2.394.53.

Macfarlane, Gwyn. *Alexander Fleming, the Man and the Myth.* Oxford University Press, 1985.

Mattern, Susan P. *The Prince of Medicine: Galen in the Roman Empire.* Oxford University Press, 2013.

McNeill, William Hardy. *History of Western Civilization: a Handbook.* University of Chicago Press, 1986.

"NLM Exhibitions and Public Programs." *U.S. National Library of Medicine*, National Institutes of Health, 24 Oct. 2006, www.nlm.nih.gov/exhibition islamic medical.

Nuland, Sherwin B. *The Doctors' Plague: Germs, Childbed Fever, and the Strange Story of Ignác Semmelweis.* W.W. Norton, 2003.

Nuland, Sherwin B. *Doctors: the Biography of Medicine.* Vintage Books, 1995.

Papanicolas, Irene, et al. "Health Care Spending in the United States and Other High-Income Countries." *Jama*, vol. 319, no. 10, 2018, p. 1024., doi:10.1001/jama.2018.1150.

Pitt, Dennis, and Jean-Michel Aubin. "Joseph Lister: Father of Modern Surgery." *Canadian Journal of Surgery*, vol. 55, no. 5, 2012, doi:10.1503/cjs.007112.

Porter, Roy, and Jeremy Farrar. *The Greatest Benefit to Mankind: a Medical History of Humanity from Antiquity to the Present.* Folio Society, 2016.

Roberts, Jennifer T. *Herodotus: a Very Short Introduction.* Oxford University Press, 2011.

Russell, Bertrand. *A History of Western Philosophy, and Its Connection with Political and Social Circumstances from the Earliest Times to the Present Day.* Simon and Schuster, 2007.

Shlaes, Amity. *Coolidge.* Harper Perennial, 2014.

Starr, Paul. *The Social Transformation of American Medicine.* Basic Books, 1982.

Steinberg, Jonathan. *Bismarck: A Life*. Oxford University Press, 2011.

Tuchman, Barbara W., and Robert K. Massie. *The Guns of August: the Outbreak of World War I*. Random House Trade Paperbacks, 2014.

Wear, A., et al. *The Medical Renaissance of the Sixteenth Century*. Cambridge University Press, 2009.

Wear, Andrew. *Knowledge and Practice in English Medicine, 1550–1680*. Cambridge University Press, 2000.

Weindling, Paul. *International Health Organisations and Movements, 1918–1939*. Cambridge Univ. Press, 2007.

Zinn, Howard, and Anthony Arnove. *A People's History of the United States*. Harper, an Imprint of HarperCollins Publishers, 2017.

About the Author

Dr. Nazari is a practicing physician, medical director at two surgery centers, and a member of faculty at University of Central Florida School of Medicine. He has travelled extensively and practiced medicine in many parts of the world, witnessing the gift and the misery of medicine. His experiences in healthcare administrative tasks and delivering care in developed and developing countries give him a unique perspective to bring the story of medicine to the audience and critically appraise the state of medicine in the United States.

Dr. Nazari has written three other books: *Lessons from East and West*, *The Great Divide*, and *The Resurgence, America in the 21st Century*.

www.ingramcontent.com/pod-product-compliance
Lightning Source LLC
Chambersburg PA
CBHW020901180526
45163CB00007B/2586